THIRD EDITION

1001
Pediatric
Treatment
Activities

Creative Ideas for Therapy Sessions

THIRD EDITION

1001
Pediatric
Treatment
Activities

Creative Ideas for Therapy Sessions

AYELET H. DANTO, MS, OTR/L

MICHELLE PRUZANSKY, MS, OTR/L

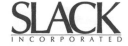

SLACK
INCORPORATED

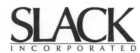

SLACK Incorporated
6900 Grove Road
Thorofare, NJ 08086 USA
856-848-1000   Fax: 856-848-6091
www.slackbooks.com
© 2023 by SLACK Incorporated

Vice President, Editorial: Jennifer Kilpatrick
Vice President, Marketing: Mary Sasso
Acquisitions Editor: Brien Cummings
Director of Editorial Operations: Jennifer Cahill
Cover: Tinhouse Design
Project Editor: Erin O'Reilly Davis

Ayelet H. Danto and *Michelle Pruzansky* reported no financial or proprietary interest in the materials presented herein.

The procedures and practices described in this publication should be implemented in a manner consistent with the professional standards set for the circumstances that apply in each specific situation. Every effort has been made to confirm the accuracy of the information presented and to correctly relate generally accepted practices. The authors, editors, and publisher cannot accept responsibility for errors or exclusions or for the outcome of the material presented herein. There is no expressed or implied warranty of this book or information imparted by it. Care has been taken to ensure that drug selection and dosages are in accordance with currently accepted/recommended practice. Off-label uses of drugs may be discussed. Due to continuing research, changes in government policy and regulations, and various effects of drug reactions and interactions, it is recommended that the reader carefully review all materials and literature provided for each drug, especially those that are new or not frequently used. Some drugs or devices in this publication have clearance for use in a restricted research setting by the Food and Drug and Administration or FDA. Each professional should determine the FDA status of any drug or device prior to use in their practice.

Any review or mention of specific companies or products is not intended as an endorsement by the author or publisher.

SLACK Incorporated uses a review process to evaluate submitted material. Prior to publication, educators or clinicians provide important feedback on the content that we publish. We welcome feedback on this work.

Library of Congress Cataloging-in-Publication Data

Names: Danto, Ayelet, author. | Pruzansky, Michelle, author.
Title: 1001 pediatric treatment activities : creative ideas for therapy
   sessions / Ayelet H. Danto, Michelle Pruzansky.
Other titles: One thousand and one pediatric treatment activities
Description: Third edition. | Thorofare, NJ : SLACK Incorporated, [2023] |
   Includes bibliographical references and index.
Identifiers: LCCN 2022030193 (print) | LCCN 2022030194 (ebook) | ISBN
   9781630919924 (spiral bound) | ISBN 9781630919931 (epub) | ISBN
   9781630919948 (PDF)
Subjects: MESH: Occupational Therapy--methods | Child | Psychomotor
   Disorders--rehabilitation | Handbook | BISAC: MEDICAL / Allied Health
   Services / Occupational Therapy
Classification: LCC RM735.3 (print) | LCC RM735.3 (ebook) | NLM WS 39 |
   DDC 615.8/515--dc23/eng/20220803
LC record available at https://lccn.loc.gov/2022030193
LC ebook record available at https://lccn.loc.gov/2022030194

Printed in the United States of America.

Last digit is print number: 10   9   8   7   6   5   4   3   2   1

DEDICATION

In loving memory of my father, Azriel Golowa A"H, and my sister Dvora Golowa A"H.
The pride they had in me has served as an inspiration.

—Ayelet

In loving memory of my grandmother Ruth Naomi Weinstein A"H,
who always took pride in her grandchildren's accomplishments.

—Michelle

CONTENTS

ACKNOWLEDGMENTS

First, I thank God for giving us the opportunity, ability, and idea to write this book.

I thank my mother, Judith Golowa, and my in-laws, Dr. Joseph and Marilyn Danto, for all their support, encouragement, and unconditional love.

To the best children a mother could want, Avraham Simcha, Moshe, Sara, Aharon, Nechama, and Racheli, I love you more than you can know.

Finally, I thank my best friend and partner in everything, my husband, Nesanel, for his endless love, constant support, and wisdom.

—Ayelet

I would like to thank my parents and in-laws, Brenda and Bill Wiener and Amy and Lawrence Pruzansky, for always supporting me, believing in me, and being there for me. Your love and guidance have meant the world to me. You are all wonderful parents and grandparents. I know I can count on you for anything in the world and am lucky to have you all in my life.

I would like to thank my children, Samantha, Ally, and Nicole. Raising three beautiful daughters, you are a constant source of love, joy, and pride.

Lastly, to my wonderful husband, Jason. You dedicate your life to your family and bring me smiles and happiness. I love you.

—Michelle

ABOUT THE AUTHORS

Ayelet H. Danto, MS, OTR/L, is an occupational therapist who has worked in various school settings with a broad range of diagnoses. She currently works in the Passaic public school system. Ayelet received her bachelor's degree in psychology from Yeshiva University Stern College for Women and a master's degree in occupational therapy from Columbia University. She resides in Passaic, New Jersey, with her husband and children.

Michelle Pruzansky, MS, OTR/L, is a pediatric occupational therapist specializing in the treatment of children with autism spectrum disorder. Michelle received her bachelor's degree from Yeshiva University Stern College for Women and her master's degree in occupational therapy from Columbia University. Michelle currently lives in New Milford, New Jersey, with her husband and children. She currently works in various school settings in New Jersey.

INTRODUCTION

As many pediatric therapists know, when working with children for extended periods of time in the same environment, it is quite challenging to find and develop new and exciting treatment activities. In order to be effective, therapists must not only treat specific impairments, but do so in a creative and resourceful manner that engages children and maintains their attention and interest. It is for this reason that we developed this guidebook.

History

While working in a public school setting in a multidisciplinary team of therapists, we found ourselves using the same activities over and over again. It became challenging for the therapists to constantly be coming up with fresh ideas. To make matters worse, many children noticed that they were engaging in the same activities session after session. Hearing "Didn't we already play this game?" or "This again?" was not encouraging. In an effort to find new ideas, we searched for different resources and books that could help with this problem. Although we were able to find some resources that addressed a specific treatment area, we were not able to find any that comprehensively covered the gamut of treatment areas that were typically addressed in a pediatric setting. So, we decided to take action and do something about this problem.

We started by putting together a list of treatment areas that are typically addressed in pediatric therapy. We then began to compile lists of different and exciting activities for each treatment area with the help of other therapists from a variety of disciplines. Every day we would add new activities to our list. This small list began to evolve into a binder full of activities. Soon enough, we started to realize that even the most creative and experienced therapist can really benefit from new ideas. That is when we decided to put our efforts toward publishing this book.

Purpose

The purpose of this book is to enhance resources available to therapists. This book serves to add to our profession's working knowledge and access to treatment activity ideas in a wide range of areas. It is meant to be a quick and simple reference or handbook for any pediatric therapist looking for new ideas for a therapy session.

How to Use This Book

As this book is intended to be used as a quick reference, it is not meant to provide a detailed activity analysis for the different topics addressed. The book was organized and written in a way that enables its user to quickly open it and skim a chapter for new ideas. The activities were carefully organized and written in simple language and with the intent of being as concise as possible.

While most activities can be explained in a short sentence, some activities require elaboration. Therefore, many activities in this book are also accompanied by a photograph to help further illustrate the intent and setup of the activity.

Contents and Organization

The information in this book is divided into eight sections, each with multiple chapters. Each chapter within a given section provides the following information:

- An introduction
- A brief description explaining the treatment topic
- An explanation of why a particular skill is important
- A list of compensatory strategies that may be employed by the child who is deficient in the particular skill
- A list of treatment ideas and activities in which to engage, in order to work on the specific treatment goal
- Examples of commercial products that can be used to address the treatment goal

Generally, treatment activities were placed in the most suitable sections; however, many activities addressed more than one goal at a time. For this reason, there were several activities that were listed in multiple sections.

Frame of Reference

Multiple frames of reference were used when compiling this book, including the biomechanical frame of reference and the sensory motor model (Giroux Bruce & Borg, 2002). The intent of this organization was to offer a wide variety of easy-to-access activities to choose from in many different areas. However, the purpose of this book is not intended to dictate the way treatment is given, but rather to provide therapists with the tools necessary to come up with different treatment activities. It is up to the treating therapist to determine the appropriate frame of reference to use with each individual child.

Who Should Use This Book

This book was written with the intent to be used primarily by pediatric occupational and physical therapists. However, this book may also be useful for teachers, psychologists, or other pediatric educators.

Many activities provided in this book require skilled and experienced knowledge of working with children and may be harmful or ineffective if used in the wrong way. Therefore, it is important that any layperson using this book consult with a physical or occupational therapist before performing any of the suggested activities. It is also crucial that any activities that are unclear be reviewed with a trained pediatric occupational or physical therapist.

Populations Intended for

This book was written to be used in a wide range of populations and pediatric settings. Specifically, these settings include a pediatric clinic, school-based setting, hospital, and home-based therapy. When writing this book, a wide variety of diagnoses and conditions were kept in mind including, but not limited to, children with fine motor and gross motor delays, traumatic injuries, congenital abnormalities, perinatal injuries, attention deficit/hyperactivity disorder, cerebral palsy, autism spectrum disorder, dyspraxia, global delays, learning disabilities, Down syndrome, and other chromosomal disorders.

About Play

As mentioned earlier, particularly when working with children with disabilities, each child displays different strengths and weaknesses and does not necessarily develop according to a defined schedule. However, it is helpful to remember the different stages of play that children normally engage in at different points of development as a reference point. This can be of assistance in choosing age/developmentally appropriate play activities for a child from the variety of play activities included in this book.

Nancy Takata developed play epochs under the leadership of Mary Reilly, the famous occupational therapist who was instrumental in developing the occupational behavior frame of reference (Parham & Fazio, 1997).

Takata's play epochs can be understood in the explanation below (ages identified are approximate; Takata, 1974):

- Sensorimotor (age 0 to 2 years): Solitary play (no peer interaction) involving motor and sensation, such as Peek-a-Boo, "Patty Cake," imitation of caregivers, container play, exploring objects, practicing new motor skills, and simple problem solving.

- Symbolic and simple constructive (age 2 to 4 years): Beginning of make-believe and pretend play, shift from solitary play to parallel play (playing side by side with peer with little or no interaction); building simple constructions that represent another object or situation; practicing climbing and running.

- Dramatic, complex constructive, and pregame (age 4 to 7 years): More social participation; associative play (participating in group with a shared activity), dramatic role-playing enacting daily experiences, social roles, fairy tales, and myths; skill in activities requiring hand dexterity; daredevil activities involving strength and skill outdoors; constructions are realistic and complex; verbal humor, creates rhymes.

- Game (age 7 to 12 years): Games with rules; fascination with rules; masters established rules and makes up new ones; risk taking in games; concern with peer status; friendship groups are important; interest in sports and formal groups; cooperative play (cooperates with peers in highly organized activity); interest in how things work, nature, and crafts.

- Recreational (age 12 to 16 years): Formal peer group orientation, teamwork, cooperation, respect for rules, games that challenge skills, competitive sports, service clubs; realistic constructive projects and complex manual skills. Although this information is helpful, when choosing a play activity for a child, it is of the utmost importance to keep in mind the preferences and desires of the particular child with whom you are working.

Final Things to Consider

- Grading: Grading an activity is the ability to modify an activity's challenge level to suit the skill level of a child. While some methods of gradation are provided within this book, it is left up to the treating therapist for the most part to properly grade the activity to an appropriate level of challenge. Grading an activity must be done on an individual basis, keeping the different components of the activity in mind, along with the different strengths and weaknesses of the child.
- Repetition: Repetitive practice of a skill helps a child improve in an area and generalize the skill to other areas. It is for this reason that multiple activities and ideas are provided for each treatment topic addressed.
- Fatigue: When supervising children engaged in different treatment activities, it is important to watch the child's level of fatigue. Pushing a child too hard can be unsafe and ineffective from a therapeutic standpoint. This is especially true for many children with low muscle tone and other medical diagnoses.

What's New

The following items have been added to the third edition of *1001 Pediatric Treatment Activities: Creative Ideas for Therapy Sessions*:

- Dozens of new fun and engaging activities
- Full-color images and additional pictures throughout to support and help explain the various activities
- Current evidence based on today's research added to each chapter introduction
- Chapter on handwriting and an appendix on teletherapy
- An up-to-date list of therapeutic apps

Conclusion

It has been both rewarding and hard work updating, editing, and expanding upon the third edition of this book. It is our hope that our fellow clinicians benefit from the activities presented and make therapy more fun for the children with whom they work. We urge readers to use caution and sound clinical reasoning when implementing the activities provided. We challenge clinicians to continuously employ innovative strategies and expand upon what we have presented in this book. We wish all therapists the best of luck in their future endeavors!

IMPORTANT WARNING AND DISCLAIMER

The authors of this book are not responsible for use or misuse of the treatment activities provided. All activities provided should be closely supervised by a trained occupational or physical therapist or be performed under the guidance of one. Before implementing any activities provided in this book, one must first check for any medical contraindications. In addition, several activities involve the use of food; it is important to check for any food allergies before using food in an activity.

It also is important to be aware of toys or objects that may pose a choking hazard to infants and small children. The general rule is that the size of the toy should not fit through a toilet paper roll, but it is best to always consult a pediatrician.

Moreover, before beginning treatment with any child, it is always important to become familiar with the child's background information, specifically that which is related to any medical conditions or diagnoses that may have accompanying contraindications or sequelae that may adversely affect a child in a specific activity or exercise.

Finally, there are many activities throughout this book that involve the use of therapeutic handling techniques. It is important that the therapist be skilled in proper handling techniques in order to safely and effectively implement the chosen activity. To become familiar with these handling techniques, the therapist should contact a trained pediatric occupational or physical therapist familiar with the specific population of interest.

I

Sensory Integration

Sensory integration is the ability of the brain and body to take in information through the senses and interpret it meaningfully (Ayres, 2005). The seven senses include vision, touch, taste, smell, hearing, the vestibular sense (movement/balance), and the proprioceptive sense (body awareness/deep pressure; Foster & Verny, 2007). Sensory integration dysfunction, sensory processing disorder, and sensory modulation disorder refer to children who demonstrate atypical responses to sensory stimuli (Koziol et al., 2011).

The Interdisciplinary Counsel of Developmental and Learning Disorders has grouped sensory modulation disorder into three categories: sensory overresponsivity, sensory underresponsivity, and sensory seeking/craving (Koziol et al., 2011). Both hyposensitivity and hypersensitivity to sensory stimulation occur in approximately 5% of children within the general population, while it is found in 40% to 80% of children with developmental disorders (Baranek, 2002). Another manifestation of sensory integration disorder is when a child's brain and body fails to interpret sensory information properly, causing the child to be clumsy and have difficulty learning new motor tasks (Ayres, 2005).

PROPRIOCEPTIVE ACTIVITIES

Proprioception is a sense that tells a person the location and orientation of their body and limbs during stationary and movement activities (Ayres, 2005, p. 41). Difficulty processing proprioceptive input is especially common in children with developmental disabilities (Blanche et al., 2012). Proprioception can be defined as the sum of neuronal inputs from the joints, ligaments, muscles, tendons, and skin, that affects motor control and may also affect other components of sensory regulation (Ayres, 1972). Deep pressure can also be a beneficial form of proprioceptive input and result in a calming and organizing effect (Grandin, 1992). The use of proprioceptive input in the form of weighted equipment can also help increase attention in children as well (Miller et al., 1999).

Proprioceptive Activities

CLEANUP/SETUP ACTIVITIES

- Child removes chairs from table and places them on top of table during cleanup.
- Child drags and rearranges small tables, desks, chairs, and other small furniture in the room.
- Child hangs up large mats or pulls them toward one side of the room.

DEEP PRESSURE ACTIVITIES

- Bear hugs: Therapist gives child a large hug, wrapping their arms all the way around the child's trunk and shoulder girdle, maintaining constant and firm pressure.
- Mummy-wrap game: Therapist wraps child tightly in a sheet, blanket, or towel. Therapist tucks the end of the material in and has child walk across the room without letting the sheet/blanket/towel fall to the ground.
- Therapist ties two children together with Lycra material and has them walk across the room together.

- Therapist massages child's back and feet.
- Vibrations: Therapist uses an Innergizer or another vibrating machine and moves it along the child's arms, legs, and back. (Figure 1-1; refer to user's manual for safety precautions and contraindications.)
- Brushing protocol: Refer to Wilbarger's brushing protocol for instructions (Wilbarger & Wilbarger, 1991).
  - Therapist brushes and provides joint compressions to child according to brushing protocol.
  - Older children can be taught to brush themselves (joint compression will require another adult; Figure 1-2).
- Joint compressions: Refer to Wilbarger's brushing protocol for instructions (Wilbarger & Wilbarger, 1991).
- Lycra swing: The material in a Lycra swing surrounds the child's body and provides deep pressure. Different Lycra swing activities include the following:
  - Therapist swings child in Lycra swing (Figure 1-3).
  - Therapist plays Peek-a-Boo with child hidden in swing.
  - Child climbs up the swing and slides down—only with long Lycra swing (Figure 1-4).

Danto, A. H., & Pruzansky, M. *1001 Pediatric Treatment Activities: Creative Ideas for Therapy Sessions, Third Edition* (pp. 3-12).

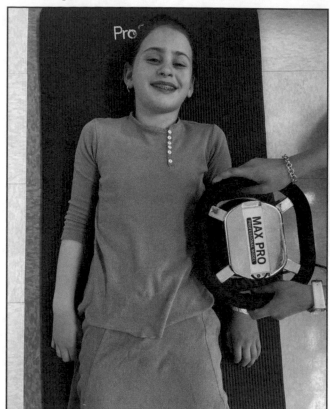

Figure 1-1.

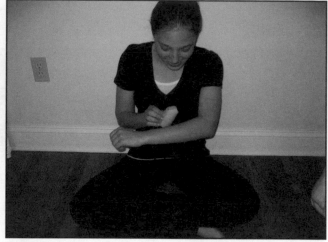

Figure 1-2.

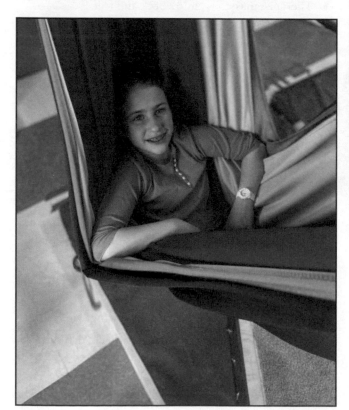

Figure 1-4.

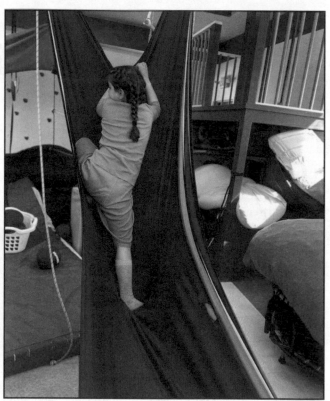

Figure 1-3.

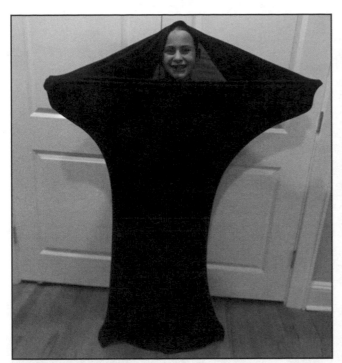

Figure 1-5.

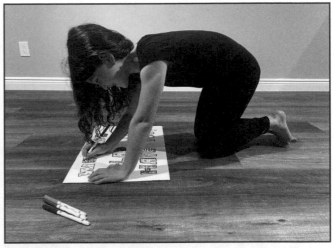

Figure 1-6.

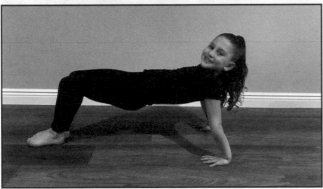

Figure 1-7.

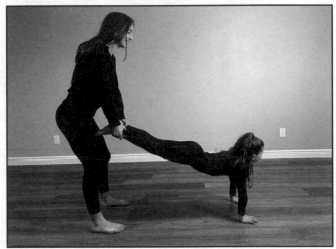

Figure 1-8.

- Body sock: Therapist places child in a body sock (Figure 1-5) and asks child to do the following:
  - Walk around the room.
  - Play Simon Says.
  - Play "Patty Cake."
- Quadruped activities: Child goes into quadruped position and does the following:
  - Colors on a large piece of oak tag (Figure 1-6).
  - Places pegs into a peg board on the floor or on a slightly raised surface.
  - Assembles a puzzle.
  - Maintains quadruped stance and counts to ten.

- Hot Dog and Sandwich games: Therapist pushes against child with big pillows and has child pretend to be a hot dog while the pillows are the buns. Therapist should use careful judgment when pushing against child and providing deep pressure.
- Ball-pit games
  - Child crashes into the ball pit.
  - Child hides self underneath the balls; then the therapist tries to find the child.
- Crab-walking: Child crab-walks across the room (Figure 1-7).
- Wheelbarrow-walking: Child wheelbarrow-walks across the room (Figure 1-8).
- Child wheelbarrow-walks up ramp and then the therapist gently pulls the child down the ramp by the legs carefully controlling the child.

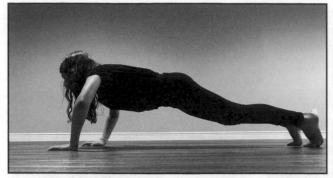

Figure 1-9.

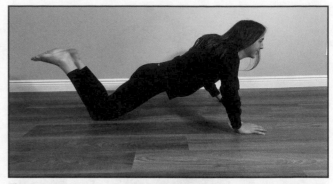

Figure 1-10.

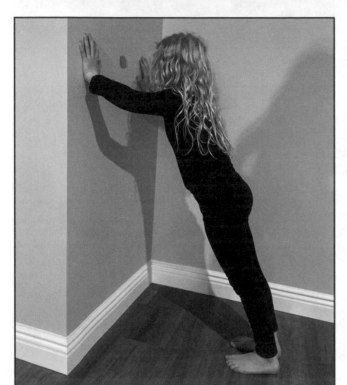

Figure 1-11.

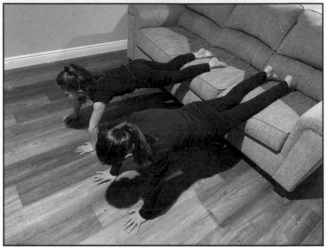

Figure 1-12.

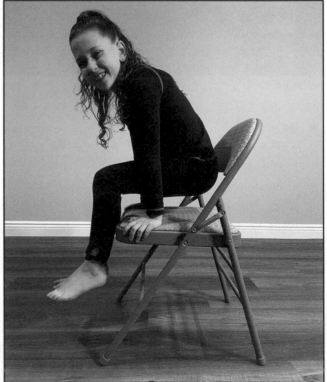

Figure 1-13.

- Push-ups: Child performs different push-ups, including
  - Regular floor push-ups (Figure 1-9).
  - Half push-ups with knees touching floor (Figure 1-10).
  - Wall push-ups (Figure 1-11).
  - Couch push-ups: Child lies on a couch on belly, hanging over the edge. Child places arms on the floor and pushes off the floor keeping lower body on the couch (Figure 1-12).
  - Chair push-ups: Child sits on a chair, grabs each side of the chair with hands and pushes down with hands in order to lift themself up slightly off the chair. The child then lowers themself back down to a seated position (Figure 1-13).

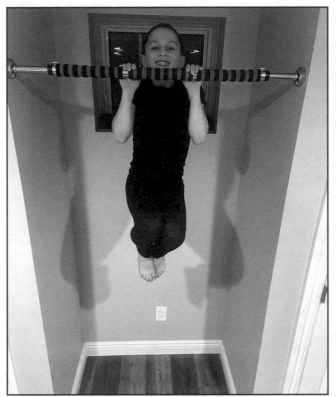

Figure 1-14.

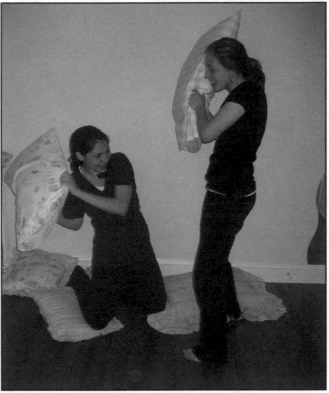

Figure 1-15.

- Chin-ups: Child pulls self up on chin-up bar (Figure 1-14).
- Controlled pillow fights: Child and therapist take turns pushing each other with large pillows. Specific rules and guidelines of this game should be made clear in advance and the game should be terminated if the child becomes too rowdy or is not following the rules (Figure 1-15).

ACTIVITIES UTILIZING WEIGHTED EQUIPMENT

Although as yet there are no standardized guidelines, many recommend that therapists should use approximately 5% of the child's total body weight when placing weights in weighted garments (Reichow et al., 2010; VandenBerg, 2001).

- Therapist places weights in child's shirt and pants pockets.

- Child wears ankle and wrist weights during an activity.
- Therapist places a weighted lap pad on child during a seated activity.
- Child wears a weighted vest.
- Child lies in prone position (on belly) and therapist places a weighted blanket over child's back.
- Child plays catch with a weighted ball.

HEAVY WORK ACTIVITIES

- Therapist places heavy objects on a scooter or in a wheelbarrow, and the child pushes it around the room.
- Therapist places several textbooks (approximately 5% of child's body weight) in child's backpack, and the child carries the heavy objects across the room.
- Therapist and child take turns giving "rides." Therapist sits on a chair with wheels and child gives a "ride." Therapist and child then switch positions, and therapist pulls child around the room.

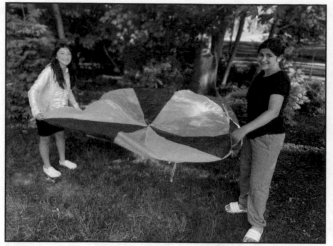

Figure 1-16.

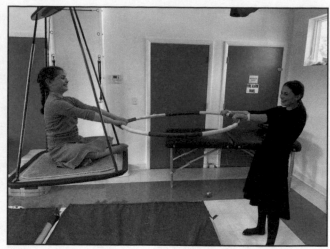

Figure 1-17.

- Parachute games: Child sits in the center of a parachute while another child pulls the parachute around with an adult assisting (Figure 1-16).
- Scooter activities
  - Child lies on belly on a scooter board and propels themself around the room using upper extremities.
  - Child lies on belly on a scooter board and pulls themself up a ramp using upper extremities.
  - Child lies on belly on a scooter board and holds onto a bungee cord or jump rope and gets pulled by therapist. (An alternative method of this game would be to have child lie in prone position on the scooter board, tie a jump rope around a doorknob, and have the child pull themself back and forth.)
  - Child and therapist make large Tic-Tac-Toe board with masking tape on the floor. Child cuts out circles and squares out of construction paper. Both then play Tic-Tac-Toe prone on scooters.
  - Therapist places Tic-Tac-Toe pieces on the other side of the room and has child use a scooter board to retrieve each piece at each turn.
- Child sits on swing and holds onto one end of a Hula Hoop. Therapist holds onto the other end and pulls child back and forth on the swing (Figure 1-17).
- Squeeze a squeeze toy: Child squeezes a resistive ball, Koosh ball, or other sensory ball.
- Velcro toys: Child pulls apart different toys fastened together by heavy-duty Velcro.
- Child pretends to be as strong as a superhero with special powers. Child then pushes against the walls and pretends that the walls are moving.

- Leaning Tower of Pisa game: Two children (or therapist and child) face each other and place hands palm-to-palm. Therapist and child lean into each other and hold this position for as long as possible, pretending to be the Leaning Tower of Pisa (Figure 1-18). This activity should be performed on a mat and closely supervised.
- Modified wrestling: Therapist faces child. Therapist and child lock hands and lean in toward each other. The object of this game is to see who can keep their balance longer without falling backward or to the side. This game should be closely supervised to make sure nobody gets hurt and should be only played with a child who will not become overly rowdy. This game should be played on a soft mat.
- "Row, Row, Row Your Boat" game: In this game, child sits on the floor, facing either the therapist or another child, each holding onto one end of a jump rope (position I) or onto each other's wrists (position II). As both sing the song, one person leans back as the other leans forward and then the opposite.
  - Position I (Figure 1-19).
  - Position II (Figure 1-20).
- Therapy ball activities
  - Therapist rolls a very large therapy ball toward the child quickly. Child must stop it and then push it back toward the therapist very hard and quickly.
  - Child pushes against a large therapy ball while another child or therapist gives resistance from the other side (Figure 1-21).

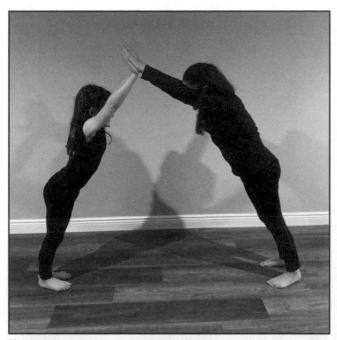

Figure 1-18.

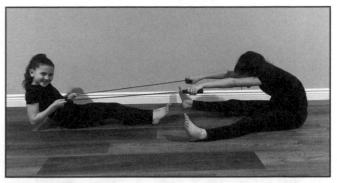

Figure 1-19.

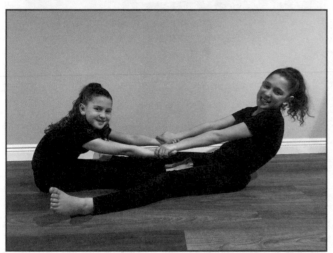

Figure 1-20.

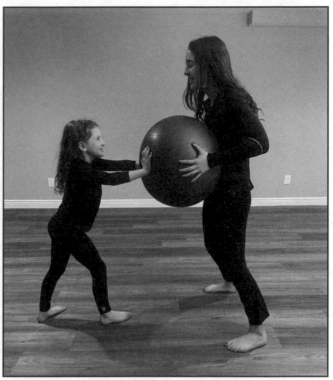

Figure 1-21.

- ○ Child pushes a large therapy ball through a Lycra tunnel. Make sure that the therapy ball is larger than the walls of the tunnel so that the child will have to use resistance to push the ball through (Figures 1-22 and 1-23).

- ○ Child holds a medium-sized therapy ball in the air with arms and legs while lying on back. Therapist tries to take the ball away and has child hold onto the ball as tightly as possible.

- Door opener: Child opens a large, heavy door and then keeps it open while others walk through.

- Bubble Wrap
  - ○ Child pops bubbles on Bubble Wrap paper.
  - ○ Child jumps up and down on a sheet of large Bubble Wrap paper.

- Stapling: Child staples papers onto a bulletin board with adult supervision or assists in stapling stacks of papers that need to be stapled together.

- Theraputty exercises
  - ○ Child pinches, pulls, and squeezes Theraputty.
  - ○ Child hides different objects in the putty and then tries to find them as quickly as possible. (This activity can be made more exciting by using a timer to see how quickly the child can work and then see if the child can break their record or by letting them keep a prize found in the putty.)

- Theraband exercises
  - ○ Child places Theraband under both feet and pulls up with both arms at each side (Figure 1-24).

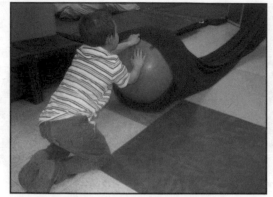

Figure 1-22.

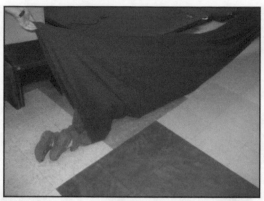

Figure 1-23.

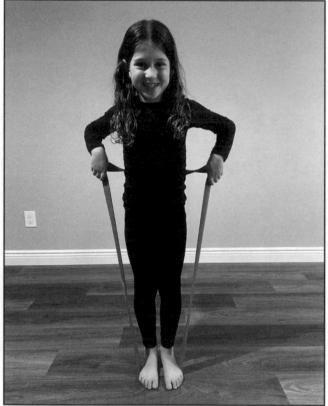

Figure 1-24.

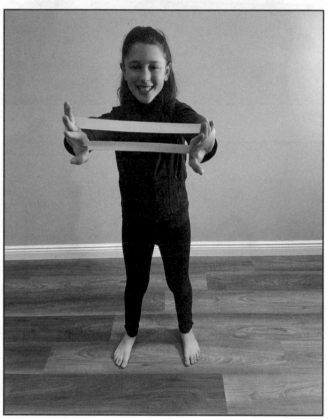

Figure 1-25.

- ○ Child holds Theraband with both hands at chest level and pulls Theraband apart to each side (Figure 1-25).

- ○ Child holds Theraband behind back and pulls out with both hands (Figure 1-26).

- ○ Therapist ties Theraband to the side of a chair. Child pulls and tugs at Theraband throughout therapy session or during class as needed while performing seated activities.

- ○ Therapist ties Theraband around both front legs of a chair and lets child kick back at Theraband as needed in the therapy session or the classroom.

- • Child colors on a chalkboard or dry-erase board and then washes and dries the board, pushing very hard onto the surface.

- • Tug-of-war (Figure 1-27).

- • Trapeze bar: Child hangs onto trapeze bar by holding on with hands or hanging upside down and hanging from legs.

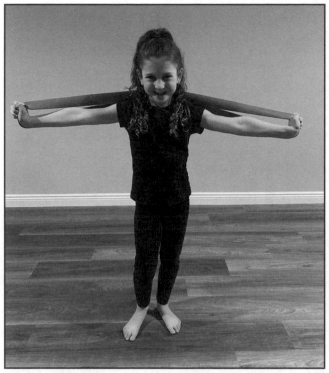

Figure 1-26.

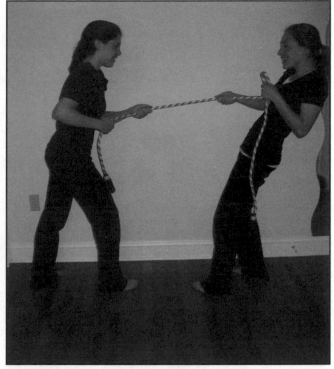

Figure 1-27.

CLIMBING ACTIVITIES

- Child climbs up a ladder in the therapy room.
- Child climbs up the wall with their legs: Place child in a quadruped position with child's feet next to the wall. Have child walk feet slowly up the wall so that the child's body is in a 90-degree angle with the wall (Figure 1-28).
- Child swings across monkey bars on the playground (Figure 1-29).
- Child hangs on single monkey bar on the playground (Figure 1-30).

JUMPING ACTIVITIES

Should be done under close supervision of a therapist.

- "Pop Goes the Weasel": Child squats on the floor and sings "Pop Goes the Weasel." Every time the word "pop" is sung, child should jump up.
- "Five Little Monkeys Jumping on a Bed": Child squats on the floor and sings "Five Little Monkeys Jumping on a Bed." The child should jump up and down during this part of the song. Child should then crash into a large pillow or bean bag at the point where the song says "one fell off and bumped his head."

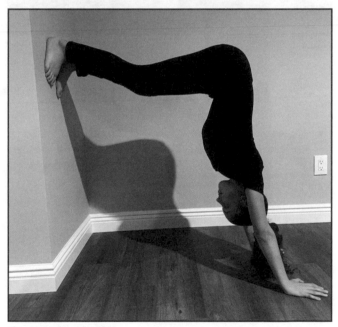

Figure 1-28.

- Relay races: Have child or group of children frog jump from one end of the room to the other.
- Child jumps on a trampoline and then crashes into big pillows.
- Child jumps up and down on either a mattress or large pillows/bean bags.
- Child jumps off of a high surface into a large bean-bag pillow.

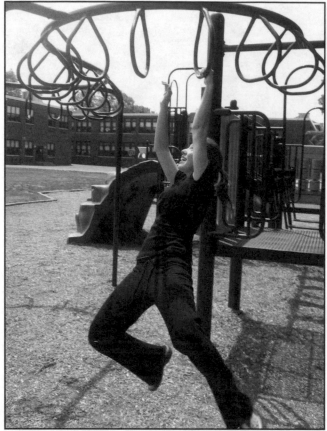

Figure 1-29.

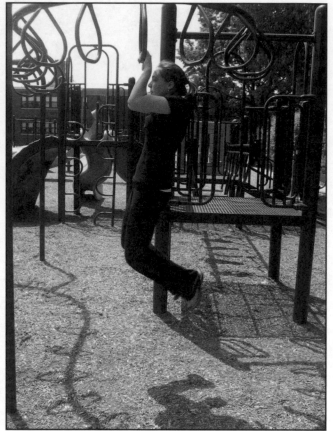

Figure 1-30.

BAKING ACTIVITIES

- Knead dough: Therapist and child perform a baking activity that requires kneading dough (e.g., cookies, pizza, bread). Child uses hands to knead the dough.

- Therapist uses a recipe that requires mixing of heavy dough or another resistive substance and has child mix the batter with a baking utensil or handheld non-electric mixer.

SPECIAL FOODS TO EAT

Be aware of any allergies or special diets before giving a child any food. Additionally, rule out any feeding or swallowing problems before using food in treatment.

- Therapist provides child with crunchy/hard foods, such as oat bars and crunchy cereal.

- Therapist provides child with chewy foods, including bagels, gum, licorice, chewy bars, and peanut butter.

Motor Planning

Motor planning refers to the process of preparation of a movement that occurs during the reaction time prior to onset of the movement (Wong et al., 2015). A child with motor planning difficulties may appear clumsy and uncoordinated. Difficulty with motor planning is often associated with decreased body awareness (Ayres, 1965). There is an association between engaging in physical exercises involving complex motor planning tasks and a neurological change in the motor pathways of the areas in the brain controlling these movements (Jacini et al., 2009). There is a long history of occupational therapy being involved in the treatment of motor coordination impairments (Wilson et al., 2000).

MOTOR PLANNING TREATMENT ACTIVITIES

Ball Activities

- Neck ball: Child holds a ball with neck and passes it along to another child's neck without using hands (Figure 2-1).

- Tic-tock-tire: Therapist hangs up a tire swing (a Hula Hoop is okay, too) and swings it from side to side. A bucket full of small items (bean bags, Koosh balls, etc.) is placed on the floor to the side of the child. The child is asked to pick up one item at a time and throw it through the moving tire without letting it touch the tire.

  - To make this activity more challenging, ask child to stand on a balance board while throwing the bean bags.

  - To downgrade this activity, keep the tire still or move it ever so slightly (Figure 2-2).

  - This activity can also be played in the form of catch, with the child standing on one side of the tire and the therapist on the other. The game is played with a small ball while keeping the tire swaying from side to side.

Body Positioning

- Imitation of different body positions

  - Child tries to imitate another child or therapist's position.

Danto, A. H., & Pruzansky, M. *1001 Pediatric Treatment Activities: Creative Ideas for Therapy Sessions, Third Edition* (pp. 13-19).
© 2023 SLACK Incorporated.

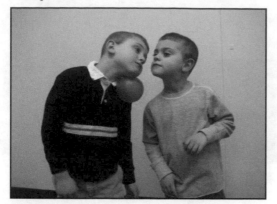

Figure 2-1.

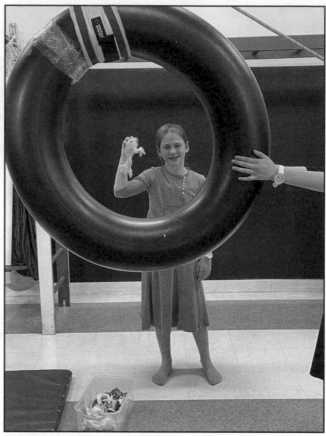

Figure 2-2.

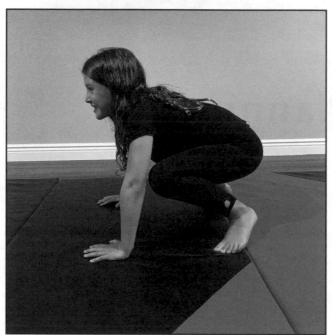

Figure 2-3.

○ Child plays Simon Says, imitating different positions.

○ Child is shown photographs of people in different positions and tries to place self in same position as person in the photograph.

- Imitation of different finger and hand positions: Therapist faces child and positions own hands or fingers in a specific position. Therapist holds the position and asks child to try to create a mirror image of the position.

- Animal-walk: Therapist assigns child an animal and then asks child to assume the different animal positions. Child then walks across room in these positions. Some examples include frog, kangaroo, snake, elephant, lion, bear, and rabbit (Figures 2-3 and 2-4).

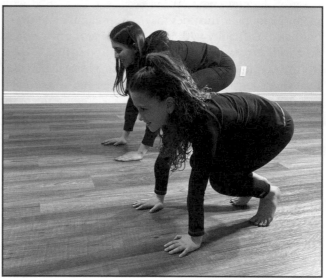

Figure 2-4.

- Statue game: This activity can be played one to one or in a group. Therapist designates a leader and asks the leader to pretend to be different statues. Child must then try to imitate the different statues and positions.

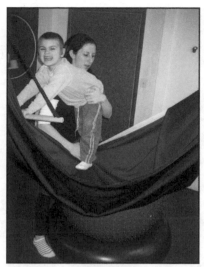

Figure 2-5.

- Body letter making: Therapist places children in groups of two to four. Therapist asks each group to pick a letter (A to Z) out of a hat. Therapist tells children in a specific group to try to place their bodies in the correct positions to make the letter on the floor. (This game can also be played individually but will then work with only some of the alphabet letters.)

Body Movement Games

- Child points to and labels different body parts upon request. This activity can be made more exciting if played to a song, such as "Head, Shoulders, Knees, and Toes" and "If You're Happy and You Know It (touch your nose, head, etc.)." (Singing these songs in front of a mirror may help if child is having trouble touching the correct body part.)

- "Hokey Pokey": Therapist sings the "Hokey Pokey" song while helping child place the correct body part in and out of the circle. (This game can also be helpful for right/left orientation.)

- Hopscotch: Therapist creates a hopscotch board on the floor with masking tape (or sidewalk chalk outside). Child plays hopscotch and concentrates, when jumping, on opening, closing, and alternating feet onto correct spaces.

- Child climbs on top of a therapy ball and uses a trapeze bar to climb into a Lycra swing. To upgrade this activity, tell the child which foot/arm to put in first (Figure 2-5).

- Elbow to knee: Child raises left knee and taps it with right elbow, then repeats on opposite knee with other hand (Figures 2-6 and 2-7).

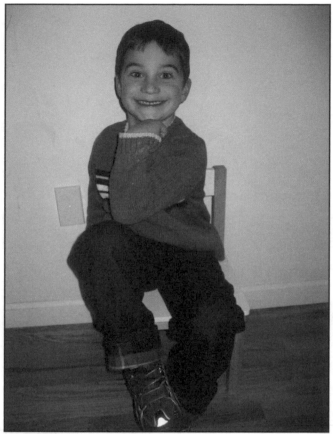

Figure 2-6.

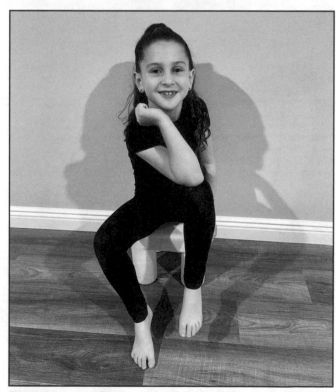

Figure 2-7.

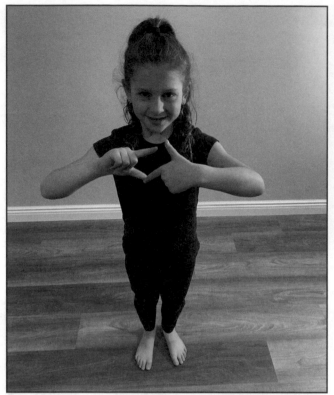

Figure 2-8.

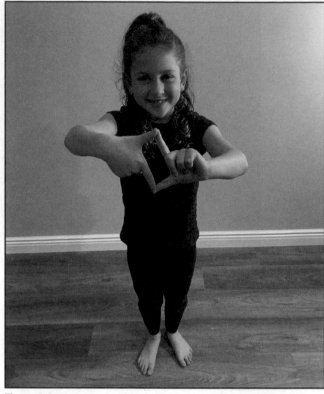

Figure 2-9.

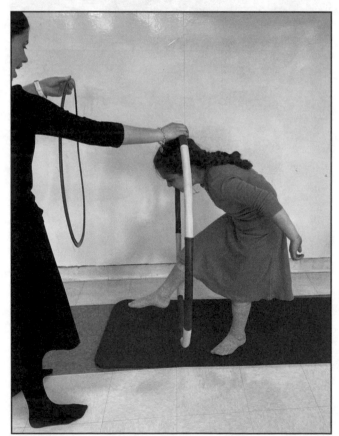

Figure 2-10.

- Child sings "The Itsy Bitsy Spider" along with therapist. Child brings right index finger to the left thumb and left index finger to the right thumb, then flips fingers up in alternating fashion (Figures 2-8 and 2-9).

- Child self-pumps on frog swing or on playground swing.

- Therapist holds up a series of Hula Hoops and child crawls/walks through them without letting the hoops touch their body. Child can also try and walk through the tire swing without touching it (Figure 2-10).

- Child spins a Hula Hoop around each wrist, starting and stopping every few seconds on cue (Figure 2-11).

- Child performs multistep obstacle courses, which can include the following:
  - Climbing toys
  - Slides
  - Crash mats
  - Bean bags
  - Ball pits
  - Balance beam/balance board
  - Trampolines
  - Suspended equipment

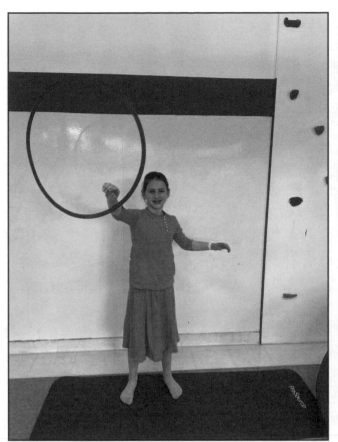

Figure 2-11.

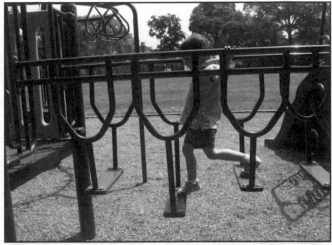

Figure 2-12.

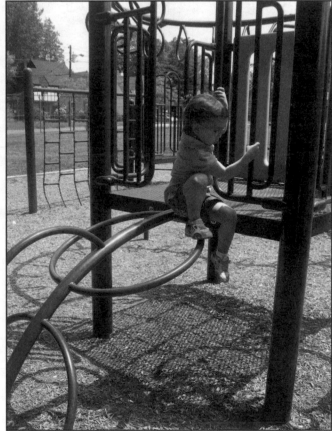

Figure 2-13.

- Child climbs on unfamiliar playground equipment (Figures 2-12 through 2-15).

- Therapist places toy a small distance from the child (developmental age 7 to 12 months; Cottrell, 2004, p. 19). While sitting on the floor, therapist then puts out his or her leg as an obstacle for the child to crawl over in order to get to the desired toy.

  ○ The therapist can also place other obstacles, such as pillows or soft wedges, for the child to crawl over.

Activities With Eyes Closed

- Child closes eyes, and therapist touches a specific body part on the child, applying consistent pressure for 1 or 2 seconds and then removing hand. Child then opens eyes and identifies the body part touched.

- Therapist places a red dot on the wall at the child's eye level. Child moves index finger from nose to dot and back three consecutive times. Child then tries to perform this activity with eyes closed.

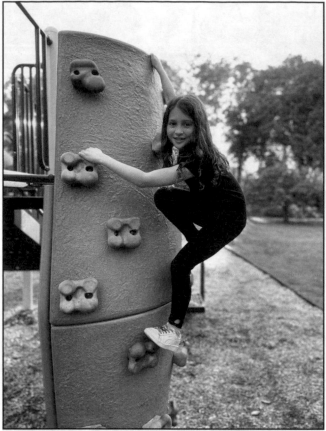

Figure 2-14.

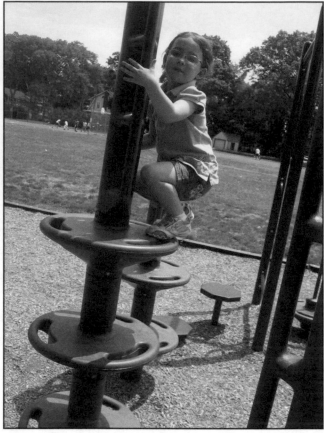

Figure 2-15.

- Therapist draws a number/letter/shape with finger on child's back. Child tries to guess what was drawn.
  - This activity can also be played on child's hands: Have child close eyes and then therapist draws a number/letter/shape on back of the child's hand. Child then guesses what was drawn.
  - This activity can be downgraded by giving child a choice of two possible guesses of things that were drawn.
- Hide and seek: Therapist and child play together. (This activity requires child to completely cover their entire body, which helps to increase awareness to all the different parts of the body. This is because the child must pay attention to body parts that are occluded from vision.)

Rolling

- Child rolls on a mat and keeps body straight.
- Log-roll game: Child rolls on mat. When therapist says stop, child must freeze and say if they are on back, belly, or side.

Running, Skipping, Jumping

- Child performs a running jump through tire swing. (A mat must be used, and the therapist should lower the swing so that the child is able to jump through easily.)
- Therapist teaches child how to skip and gallop.
- Child practices jumping rope (Figure 2-16).

Commercially Available Products

- First Hand
- Jenga
- Skip It
- Twister
- Woggler

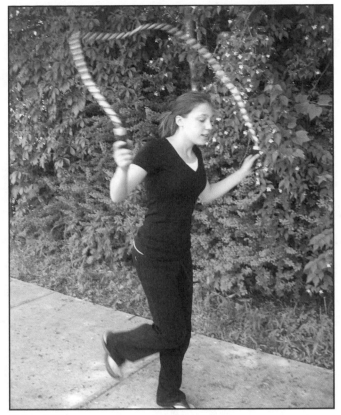

Figure 2-16.

3

Pressure Modulation

Pressure modulation is the ability of the body and joints to know the level of force to exert when completing a motor task. Poor pressure modulation can occur in many areas, from self-care to play activities. For example, a child with decreased pressure modulation may be unable to push toys together or pull them apart. Using too much or too little force during writing tasks is a common problem faced by many children (Srivastava, 2016). Research has shown a relationship between high pressure or force on a writing instrument associated with decreased legibility (Harris & Rarick, 1959). Inability to grade force may even have social implications, as a child may unknowingly be overly aggressive with their peers.

There are many activities and exercises that can help a child improve pressure modulation. Activities that combine discrimination of tactile, proprioceptive, and vestibular components can lead to smooth, graded, and coordinated movement (Miller et al., 2007). The exercises provided in this chapter require a child to grade their force in order to be successful with that activity. When performing an activity requiring the use of graded force, a therapist can upgrade the activity by placing a balance demand on the child in addition to the pressure modulation exercise itself. This will additionally challenge the child because this activity requires more refined and precise pressure grading when placed on dynamic surfaces or during movement activities.

PRESSURE MODULATION ACTIVITIES

Sports

There are several sports that require precise pressure modulation in order to be played successfully. Some of these include basketball, volleyball, miniature golf, ping-pong, and billiards/pool.

- Child throws a ball against the wall and catches it. (Upgrade this activity by having child stand on a balance beam when throwing the ball.)

- Child throws a ball to a Velcro bull's-eye target (Figure 3-1).

- Balloon volleyball: Child hits balloon toward therapist with either a racquet or hands. Child tries to keep balloon from touching the floor as long as possible.

- Horseshoe toss: Therapist places stakes or sticks onto the floor or in the ground outside. Therapist provides child with horseshoes and has child toss the horseshoes onto the sticks.

Danto, A. H., & Pruzansky, M. *1001 Pediatric Treatment Activities: Creative Ideas for Therapy Sessions, Third Edition* (pp. 21-24). © 2023 SLACK Incorporated.

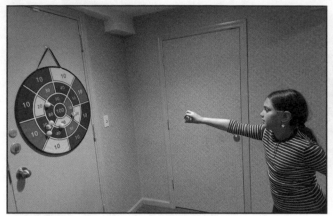

Figure 3-1.

- Ring toss: Therapist places cones on floor and provides child with rings or Hula Hoops. Child then tosses rings onto cones.
- Darts: Child shoots darts onto wall or a bull's-eye. (The child can stand further or closer to the wall in order to upgrade or downgrade the activity.)
- Skee-Ball: Child plays Skee-Ball if the equipment is available or therapist can simulate a Skee-Ball setup.

Craft Projects

- Rainbow making: Therapist gives each child a black-and-white rainbow. (See p. 192 of Appendix A for sample template of project.) Child squeezes glue onto one line at a time and then sprinkles glitter on that line. Child proceeds to glue the following line and sprinkle it with glitter of a different color.
- Puff paint: Child creates craft projects using puff paint. Therapist reminds child that if too much pressure is applied to the tube, too much paint may come out.
- Tinfoil writing: Child writes name or makes a picture with toothpicks on a piece of tinfoil and tries not to rip the foil.
- Therapist places piece of paper on a soft surface (e.g., cushioned chair, mouse pad) and provides child with sharpened pencil (pencil tip must be very pointy). Child then writes on paper or colors picture on paper without poking hole through paper.
- Glitter-glue pens: Child squeezes pens to make a picture.

Shading and Rubbing Projects

- Coin shading: Child places a quarter or another coin under a piece of thin, white paper (not construction paper). Therapist provides child with a pencil and child lightly rubs pencil over the paper on top of the coin. A light imprint of the coin should show up on the paper.

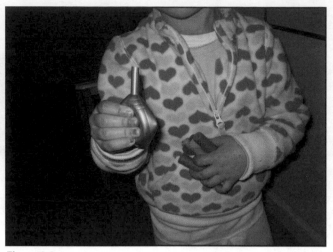

Figure 3-2.

- Letter/shape shading: Therapist places cutout letters or other shapes from poster board and places them under the paper and asks child to shade the paper with a pencil or crayon.
- Leaf shading: Therapist places leaves under a piece of thin, white paper and asks child to lightly shade on top of the paper with a pencil or crayons.

Picture Making

- Child draws the same picture three times with either a crayon or a pencil. The first time the child should draw it as hard as possible, the second time as soft as possible, and the third time with a middle amount of pressure. For smaller children who cannot understand this task, ask them to just draw three lines (hard, soft, and medium).

Cookie Decorating

- Child squeezes icing onto cookies in order to decorate them.

Recreational Children's Games

- Squeeze toys: Child squeezes a rocket launcher toy toward a target on the floor (Figures 3-2 through 3-4).
- Pop Beads: Child pushes together and pulls apart Pop Beads.
- Child builds a tower with wooden blocks, trying not to allow the tower to fall.

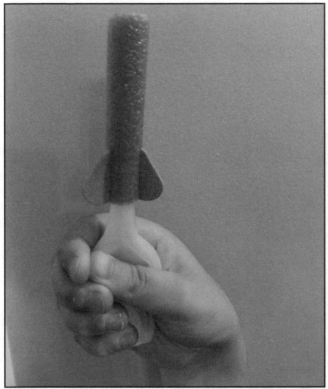

Figure 3-3.

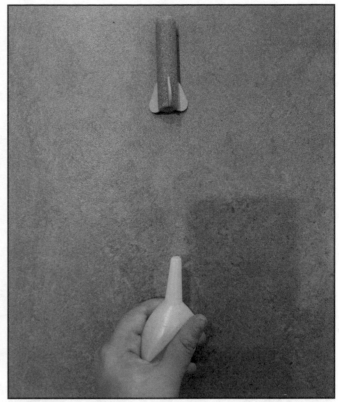

Figure 3-4.

- Dominoes: Child creates a long line of dominoes on a flat surface and then tips the last domino to watch the domino effect. It may be necessary to assist child in this task to make sure they do not accidentally knock over a domino too early (Figures 3-5 through 3-7).

- Card stacking: Child copies different card-stacking houses from a model. (An easier version of this activity is building houses or pyramids by stacking disposable plastic cups.)

- Child builds multiple stacks of 10 to 15 pennies side by side.

- Mummy-wrapping game: Child wraps another child or adult with toilet paper. Child must use only light pressure in playing this game or else the toilet paper will rip. (Try to use heavy-duty toilet paper for this project.)

- Bowling pins: Child sets up bowling pins or other light objects flat on the floor or makes a tower with them. Child then crashes into it or rolls a ball into it.

- Yo-yos: Therapist teaches child how to play with a yo-yo.

- Keyboard typing: Child types different words or plays different games on a computer keyboard.

- Lining up figurines: Child lines up small figurines gently, trying not to let them fall.

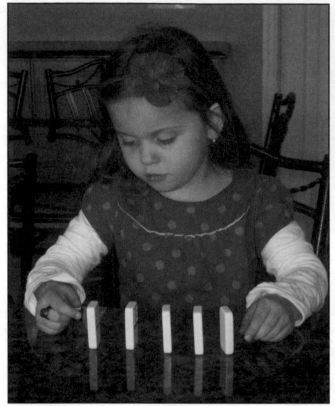

Figure 3-5.

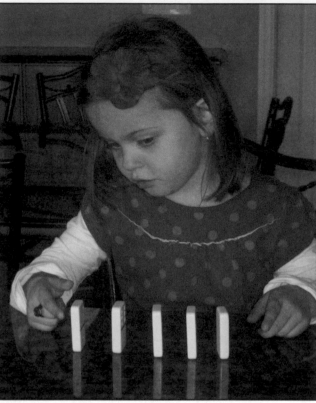

Figure 3-6.

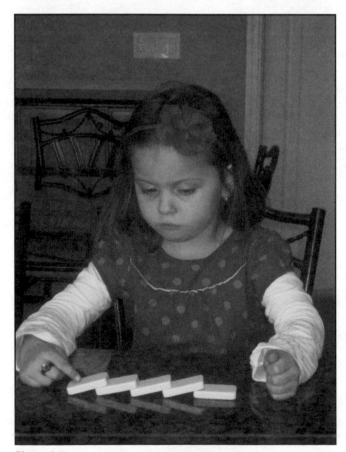

Figure 3-7.

Commercially Available Products

- Angry Birds Mega Smash
- Barrel of Monkeys
- Don't Break the Ice
- Don't Spill the Beans
- Jenga
- Kerplunk
- Konexi
- Magformers
- Magna-Tiles
- Penguin Pile-Up
- Pick Up Sticks
- Rainbow Loom
- Super Catch
- Topple Chrome

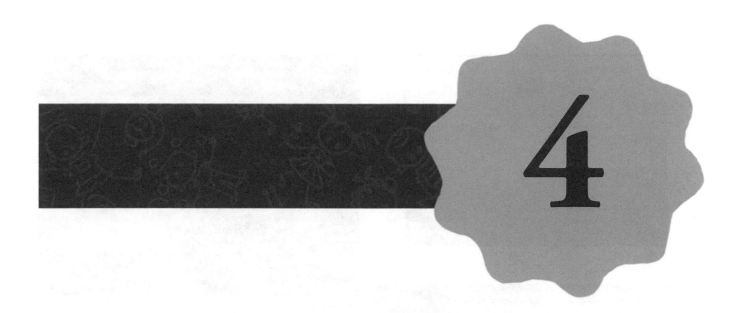

Bilateral Integration/ Crossing Midline

Bilateral integration is the ability to coordinate both sides of the body for a purposeful action. Deficits with bilateral integration can make simple, every day preschool activities challenging and frustrating (Dunbar, 1999). There are different components to bilateral integration. It includes performing an act with both sides of the body simultaneously. This is called *symmetrical bilateral integration* (e.g., rolling Play-Doh with a rolling pin, clapping hands). It also refers to using both sides of the body reciprocally, as in alternating movements (e.g., climbing stairs). Finally, bilateral integration includes using each side of the body for a different action simultaneously. This is called *asymmetrical bilateral integration* (e.g., stabilizing a paper with one hand while writing with the other, holding a jar with one hand while unscrewing the cover with the other).

Midline is a vertical line down the middle of one's body. Crossing midline means using a body part in the contralateral space (Cermak et al., 1980). An example of crossing midline would be reaching for a puzzle piece with one's right hand when the piece is placed on the left side of one's body. The ability to cross the midline is related to how well both sides of the body have become integrated and the ability to cross the midline is necessary in order for one hand to develop hand dominance (Cermak et al., 1980).

Bilateral integration and crossing midline support a child's development of fine motor skills, academic skills, and functional skills. It is needed for many everyday activities (e.g., dressing, putting on socks, turning the steering wheel when driving a car, writing across a page, many play activities; Van Hof et al., 2002).

To be able to cross midline, one needs adequate bilateral integration skills. Many activities that involve crossing midline also require the use of both hands and sides of the body simultaneously. One could say that bilateral integration and crossing midline "go hand in hand." It is for this reason that crossing midline and bilateral integration activities were put into the same section.

In working with a child with poor bilateral integration skills, it is important to be aware of the ways in which children will compensate for this deficit. Although a child may show a right-hand preference, this child will reach for objects on their left side with the left hand and transfer the object into the right hand in order to avoid crossing midline.

In setting up a therapeutic activity, it can be helpful to remind the child to use their dominant hand to pick up objects regardless of the location of the object (i.e., whether the object is to the left or right of the child). This will help to remind the child to cross midline. Many times a child will still avoid crossing midline by moving the direction of their trunk in order to face the object. It is important to help such a child stabilize the trunk when reaching, thereby forcing the child to cross midline.

Danto, A. H., & Pruzansky, M. *1001 Pediatric Treatment Activities: Creative Ideas for Therapy Sessions, Third Edition* (pp. 25-33). © 2023 SLACK Incorporated.

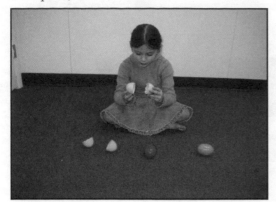

Figure 4-1.

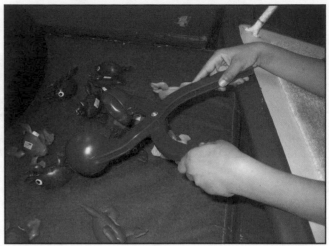

Figure 4-2.

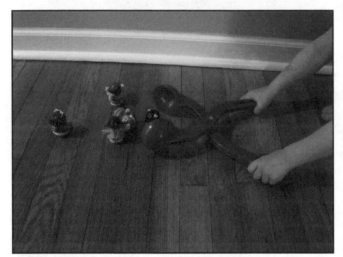

Figure 4-3.

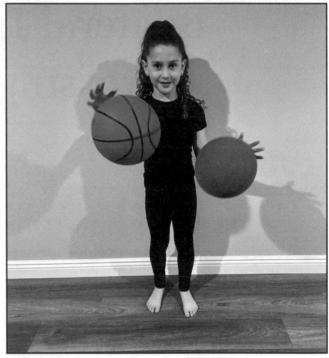

Figure 4-4.

BILATERAL INTEGRATION/ CROSSING MIDLINE TREATMENT ACTIVITIES

Symmetrical Bilateral Integration

- LEGO pieces: Child plays with LEGO pieces, pushing together pieces and pulling them apart.
- Play-Doh: Child plays with Play-Doh, rolls it, flattens it, makes a ball with it, and uses Play-Doh toys and accessories. (The therapist should encourage the child to use both hands during this activity.)
- Theraputty: Child pulls and pushes Theraputty.
- Child pushes together/pulls apart toys such as pegs or Pop Beads.

- Child opens and closes plastic eggs (Figure 4-1).
- Snow baller: Child uses a snow baller to pick toys off the floor (Figures 4-2 and 4-3).
  - Upgrade this activity by placing the child on a balance beam or on suspended equipment in using the snow baller to pick up the toys.
- Dribbling games: Child dribbles a basketball in each hand at the same time (Figure 4-4).
- Rapper Snappers: Child pulls apart/pushes together accordion plastics (Figures 4-5 and 4-6).

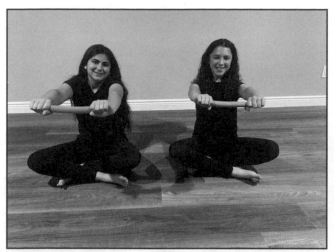

Figure 4-5.

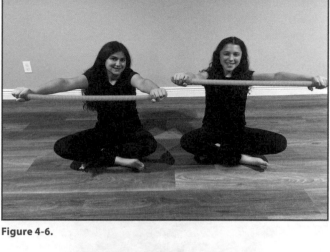

Figure 4-6.

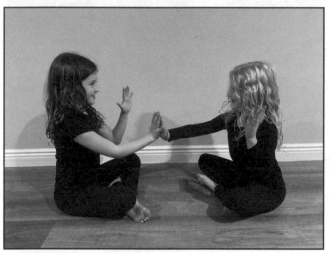

Figure 4-7.

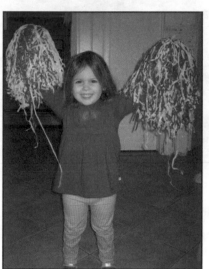

Figure 4-8.

Crossing Midline

In order to help a child become more aware of their midline while practicing crossing midline activities, place painter's tape in a vertical line on the midline of the child's trunk.

- Children's clapping games: Child 1 faces child 2. Both children claps hands together then clap alternate hand on opposite child (child 1's right hand hits child 2's right hand) and then repeats with other hand. Some games include the following:
  - "Miss Mary Mack"
  - "Patty Cake" (Figure 4-7)
- Cheerleading games: Therapist gives child pom-poms and has child watch therapist in order to imitate various cheers. Cheers should include crossing midline and using both arms together (Figures 4-8 and 4-9).

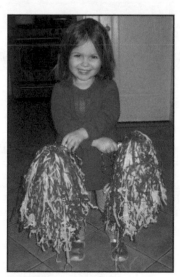

Figure 4-9.

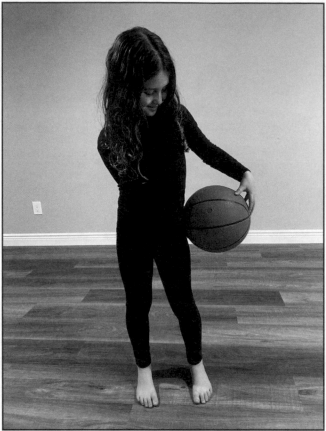

Figure 4-10.

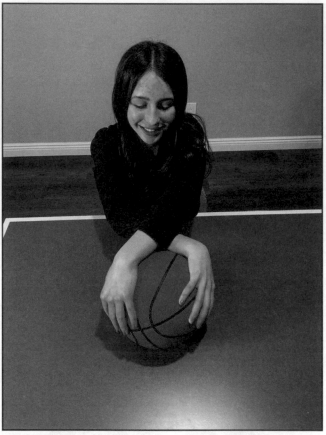

Figure 4-11.

- Stretching
  - Child stands up and brings one hand to opposite foot and switches. Repeat as tolerated.
  - Child sits in a chair and brings one elbow to the opposite knee and then switches and repeats activity as tolerated.
- Figure eights
  - Therapist tapes a large figure eight on floor. Child walks in a figure eight-style over tape.
  - Child traces large, horizontal figure eights on a piece of paper.
  - Child traces large, horizontal figure eights on a chalkboard and continues going around the figure several times.
- Therapist places balance beam on floor. Child stands to the left of the balance beam placed on the floor. Child crosses outside leg (left leg) over balance beam onto the floor while walking forward. Child then crosses outside leg (right leg) over balance beam. Child continues "criss-crossing" legs over balance beam until the end.

- Child holds a basketball and moves it in a circle around stomach, back, and back to the front (Figure 4-10).
- Child pretends to drive a car using a ball as the steering wheel. Therapist encourages child to cross hand over hand in turning the steering wheel (Figure 4-11).
- Dancing Activities:
  - Therapist puts on music with a marching beat. Child marches around room with right knee touching left elbow and left knee touching right elbow.
  - Child dances with scarves, making figure eights with arms while waving the scarves.
- Therapist places young child (developmental age of 3 to 9 months approximately) in supine position on play mat with hanging toys and encourages them to swat/reach for toys on both sides (Figure 4-12).
- Therapist places child in upright sitting position with toys placed within reach on both sides and encourages them to reach for toys on both sides (Figure 4-13).

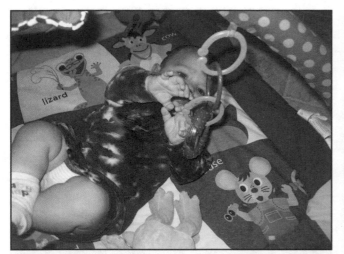

Figure 4-12.

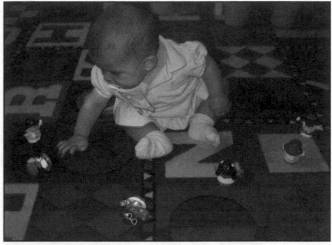

Figure 4-13.

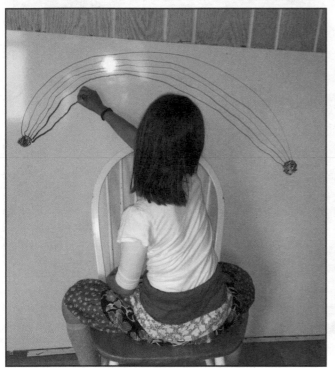

Figure 4-14.

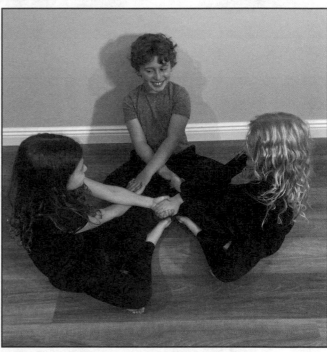

Figure 4-15.

- Child sits backward on a chair in front of an oversized paper taped to the wall or a whiteboard. (Sitting backward prevents unwanted rotation during this activity.) Therapist draws a black dot on the far left side and on the far right side of the paper with the child seated right in the middle. (Make sure child can reach each dot with dominant hand.) Using different colored crayons or markers, child draws a rainbow starting at the left dot and ending at the right dot, using dominant hand (Figure 4-14; make sure child does not switch hands being used in middle of the rainbow.)

○ Child plays game with other children where hands cross midline to clasp (Figure 4-15) and then subsequently reach up (Figure 4-16). Repeat multiple times or play singing to a song.

○ Child does push-ups facing another child. Children cross midline to "slap 5" and then repeat with other hand (Figures 4-17 and 4-18).

○ Child stands back to back with another child and passes a ball from side to side (Figures 4-19 and 4-20).

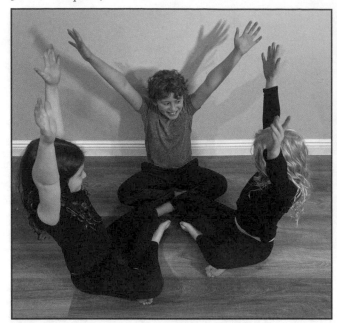

Figure 4-16.

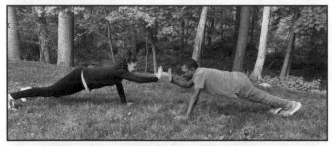

Figure 4-18.

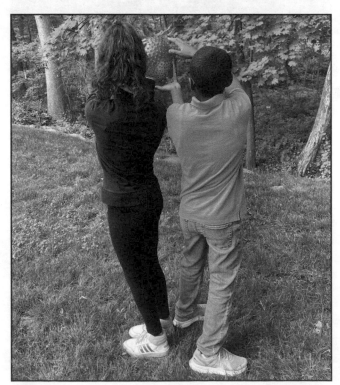

Figure 4-20.

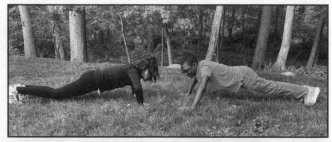

Figure 4-17.

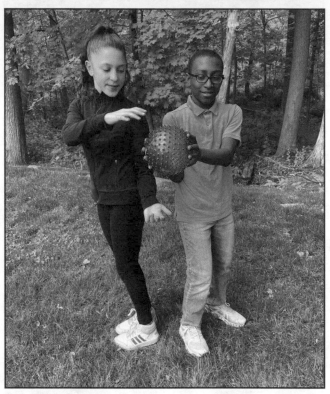

Figure 4-19.

Reciprocal Hand Use

- Child performs jumping jacks.
- Bicycle sit-ups: Child lies on back and brings the right elbow to the left knee while extending the right leg, then switches and repeats as tolerated (Figure 4-21).
- Climbing: Child climbs up a ladder or climbs up a flight of stairs on their hands.
- Double Dutch jump rope: Child tries to swing two jump ropes at a time in the Double Dutch style.
- Juggling: Therapist teaches child how to juggle two or more balls (Figure 4-22). Juggling with scarves or weighted bean bags may be a little easier than juggling balls.

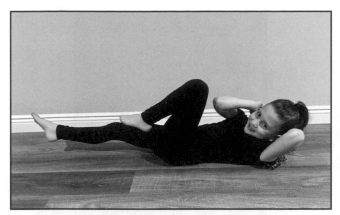

Figure 4-21.

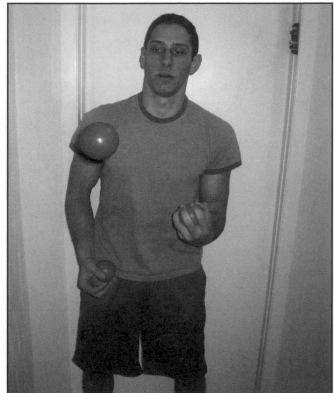

Figure 4-22.

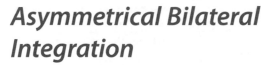

Figure 4-23.

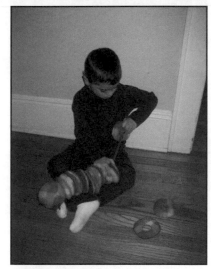

Figure 4-24.

Asymmetrical Bilateral Integration

- Lacing beads: Child holds string in one hand and a bead in the other. Child uses both hands to lace bead onto string.
- Child opens and closes jars.
- Child screws and unscrews nuts and bolts.
- Cutting activities: Child cuts strips of paper, shapes, or diagrams. (See Appendix A, pp. 193-202, for sample cutting activities.)
- Paper ring project: Child cuts out multiple strips of paper. Child glues the ends of one strip together to make a ring. Child then loops the additional strips of paper, one at a time, around the initial ring to add on more rings. Child glues the ends together, and keeps adding more rings to make a chain of paper rings (Figure 4-23).
- Lacing cards: Child uses lacing cards to lace a string in and out of the holes with one hand while stabilizing the lacing card with the other hand. (Lacing cards/boards can be created by laminating a small piece of construction paper and punching holes approximately 1 inch apart around the perimeter of the laminated paper.)

- Therapist gives child a sandwich cookie, for a snack, to break open in halves.
- Braiding: Child practices braiding on either hair, on dolls, or with pipe cleaners.
- Caterpillar toy: Pull rings off/put rings on (Figure 4-24).
- Paper airplane making: Therapist teaches child how to make paper airplanes. Therapist performs each step separately and slowly. After each step, therapist waits until child is caught up. Therapist assists child to make sure that the folding is performed accurately.

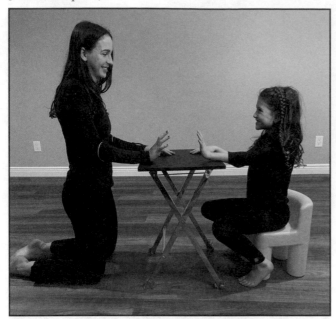

Figure 4-25.

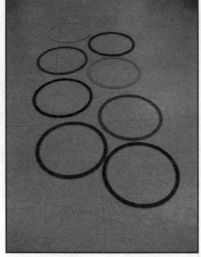

Figure 4-26.

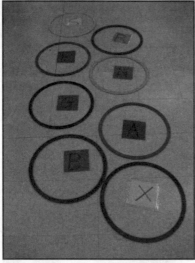

Figure 4-27.

- Table tapping: Therapist sits facing child and places both of their hands and the child's hands on the desk. One person starts by tapping the desk once with one hand. The four hands on the desk surface should try and tap the desk, one hand at a time, in a clockwise fashion. If someone taps twice in a row quickly, that alternates the direction of the circle to counterclockwise (Figure 4-25).

- Hoop jumping: Therapist places different colored hoops on the floor (Figure 4-26). Child alternates stepping into each hoop with feet and calls out the color of the hoop as the foot steps down into it. To upgrade this activity, place pictures of different letters inside the hoops and have child call out the letter in the hoop (Figure 4-27). Place pictures of animals in the hoops and have child call out name of animal (Figure 4-28).

- Knitting activities (Figure 4-29).

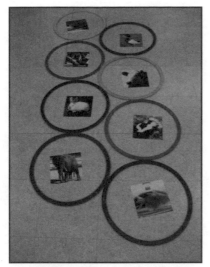

Figure 4-28.

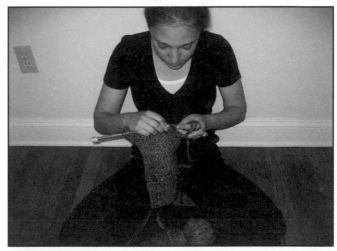

Figure 4-29.

Commercially Available Products

- Etch A Sketch
- KID K'NEX
- Mr. Potato Head
- Oreo Matchin' Middles
- Pop Beads
- Smart Snacks Sorting Shapes Cupcakes
- Twister
- Velcro fruit
- Zoom Ball

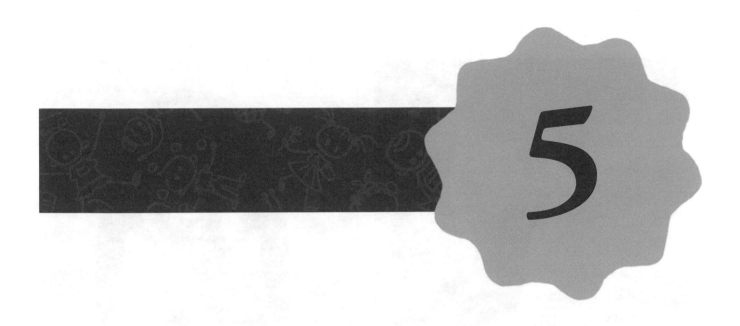

Vestibular System

The vestibular system controls a person's sense of movement, how one tolerates changes in movement, and the sense of balance. There is an increase in the reporting of vestibular deficits in children (Rine, 2009). The vestibular system is controlled by small receptors in the ears, which send messages to the brain in order to interpret movement (Ayres, 2005). Therefore changes in head position have a great impact on the vestibular system. Many children with sensory processing difficulties will have irregularities in their vestibular system. These children will be either over-responsive or underresponsive to movement.

Ayres (1979) discusses certain children who are overresponsive to movement as having "gravitational insecurity." These children will become stressed or even fear movement or being placed in specific positions. Helping regulate the vestibular system can provide a "gravitational security," which can help strengthen a child's emotional well-being (Schaft & Roley, 2006). Conversely, some children will seek increased vestibular input in a attempt to meet a high threshold of response to sensory stimuli or to gain more information from the environment (Dunn, 2001).

Research has shown that vestibular rehabilitation including balance exercises and different head movements can be effective in improving functional motor skills and independence in activities of daily living (Cohen, 1992). Vestibular rehabilitation and exercises can also be an effective tool at improving balance (Horak et al., 1992). Ongoing observation of the child and watching for various signs and symptoms is crucial in order to implement the appropriate interventions (Rine & Wiener-Vacher, 2013).

The following basic principles of the vestibular system should be reviewed before any vestibular activities are undertaken:

- Speed of movement: Different children will respond differently to different speeds of movement. Although fast movement may be more intense for some children, slow movement can be just as powerful and intense depending on the child and how an activity is set up (Ayres, 2005, p. 42).

- Length of time: The longer a child is engaged in a vestibular activity, the more intense the input will be.

- Having a child close their eyes increases the intensity of the movement provided.

- Rotary movement (spinning) can be more intense, arousing, and stimulating.

- Linear movement (back and forth) may create a more calming and organizing effect.

- A child's physical position will affect the intensity of the input. Having a child sit upright is less intense than having a child lie on their back or side (Ayres, 2005, p. 42).

Danto, A. H., & Pruzansky, M. *1001 Pediatric Treatment Activities: Creative Ideas for Therapy Sessions, Third Edition* (pp. 35-39).
© 2023 SLACK Incorporated.

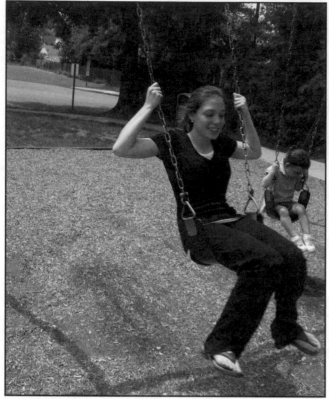

Figure 5-1.

It is important to look for signs of nausea and dizziness when engaging in movement activities. If a child becomes nauseous during an activity, stop immediately. It may also help to follow up with a proprioceptive activity in the form of deep pressure. This may help provide the child with a grounded feeling and decrease the level of nausea. (It is ideal to avoid having the child reach the point of nausea.)

Before selecting or implementing any movement activities, it is important to first review these ideas with an occupational therapist.

ACTIVITIES TO STRENGTHEN THE VESTIBULAR SYSTEM

Swinging

- Child sits/kneels/stands on different suspended equipment and swings: Allow child to place feet on floor at first, then attempt to swing child with feet off the floor.
- Child swings on an outdoor hammock.
- Child swings on a swing set swing (Figure 5-1).

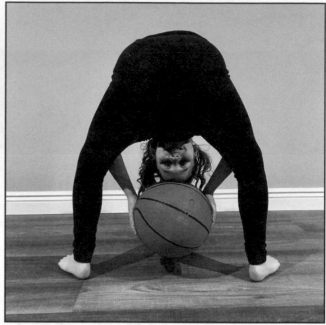

Figure 5-2.

Changing Head Positions

- Therapist slowly moves child's head in different planes of movement including to the side, backward, and forward.
- Child bends down and looks under legs and waves hello to therapist.
- Child bends down and throws a ball between legs to therapist (Figure 5-2).

Slow, Controlled Movement

- Therapist slowly rocks child in different planes on rocker chair.
- Child slowly walks up and down ramp.
- Musical Chairs: Child walks around a set of chairs and, when the music stops, the child has to sit down in one of the chairs.
- Balance beam activities
  - Child walks across a balance beam backward and forward.
  - Child walks across with eyes closed.
- Balance board activities
  - Child bends down to pick up toys off floor, then throws toys into a container/basket (Figure 5-3).
  - Child steps up onto balance board.
  - Child makes a 360-degree turn in place while standing on balance board.

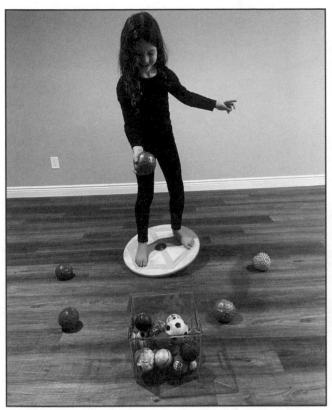

Figure 5-3.

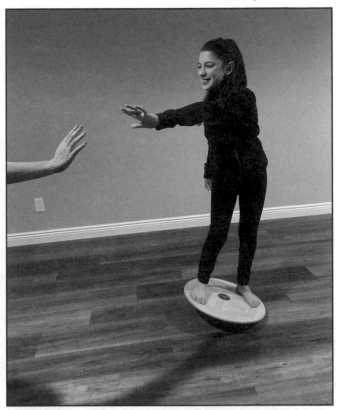

Figure 5-4.

- ○ Child slaps hands with therapist in different directional planes (Figure 5-4).
- ○ Child pops bubbles all around (Figure 5-5).
- ○ Child plays catch.
- ○ Child shoots basketballs.
- Child slowly walks up and down a flight of stairs, alternating feet when ascending or descending (instead of a step-to-step pattern). Subsequently, child attempts to do this without holding onto the railing (therapist should guard child for safety).
- Roly-poly game: Child lies on a mat and slowly rolls from one end to the other. This can be made into a game with a group of children. Designate one child as the leader who determines in which direction to roll, when to start, and when to stop. The object of the game is to avoid bumping into anyone else on the mat.
- Child goes inside a barrel. Therapist slowly rolls child across the room.
- Child sits on a swivel chair and is slowly spun around in both directions. Note: spinning needs to be controlled and monitored so as not to cause adverse effects. The child should be spun no more than 10 times in each direction at one spin/revolution per second.

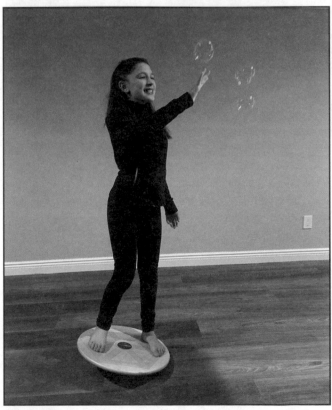

Figure 5-5.

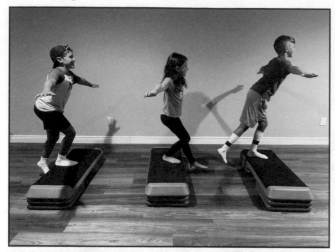

Figure 5-6.

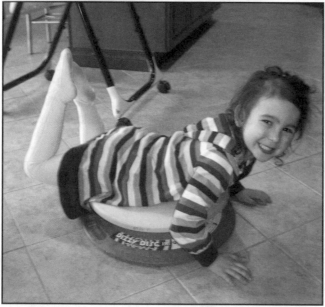

Figure 5-8.

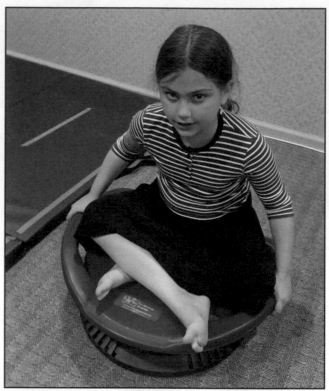

Figure 5-7.

Fast-Paced Input

- Therapy ball
  - Therapist bounces child while the child is sitting on the ball and then tips the child from side to side.
  - Therapist places child in prone position (on the belly) on the ball and then tips the child forward and to the sides (Figure 5-9).
- Hippity Hop: Child bounces across the room on a Hippity Hop toy (Figure 5-10).
- Child slides down slides of varying heights and turns.
- Two children go on a seesaw, one at each end. The children alternate between going up and down.
- Child sits on a scooter while being carefully spun around several times by therapist, as tolerated.
- Trampoline games
  - Child jumps on a trampoline and counts to 10.
  - Child runs in place on the trampoline.
  - Child sits on the trampoline and tries to bounce up and down by moving body to create momentum.
- Tag: Child plays tag or another fast-moving chasing game.

- Child climbs over big pillows and bolsters or any uneven surface.
- Child walks up onto a small, raised surface and then slowly steps down (Figure 5-6). Alternatively, child can jump down.
- "Ring Around the Rosie": Children hold hands with therapist or other children and slowly move around in a circle singing "Ring Around the Rosie."
- Somersaults: Child performs somersaults on a mat on the floor.
- Child sits on Dizzy Disc with legs crossed and is spun around or they can lie on belly on Dizzy Disc and use hands to spin self around in circles (Figures 5-7 and 5-8). Note: The child should not be spun more than 10 times in each direction at the rate of one spin per second.

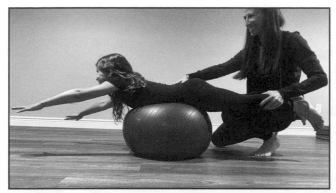

Figure 5-9.

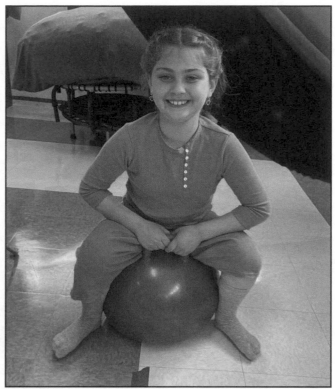

Figure 5-10.

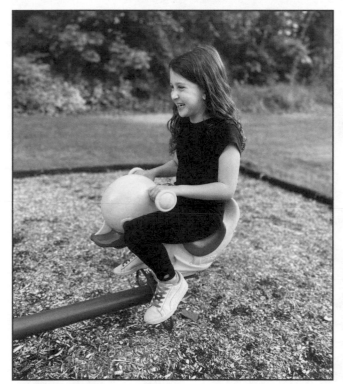

Figure 5-11.

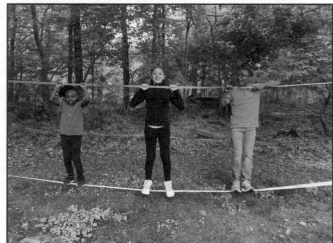

Figure 5-12.

- Jumping off surfaces of varying heights: Child holds hands with therapist and jumps in the air off of the floor. Child then jumps off a slightly higher surface. Therapist should continue raising the height of the surface slightly. If at any point the child is fearful, allow child to hold both of the therapist's hands or fingers. Provide child with as minimal physical assistance as possible.

- Child quickly walks up and down a flight of stairs, alternating feet (instead of step-to-step pattern). Subsequently, child attempts to do this without holding onto the railing. Therapist should closely and carefully guard for safety.

- Child sits on a swivel chair and is quickly spun around in both directions.

- Chair rides: Child sits on a chair with wheels. Therapist quickly pulls child around the room on chair.

- Child rocks back and forth on rocking playground toys (Figure 5-11).

- Children bounce up and down on any outdoor slack line or bungee rope (Figure 5-12).

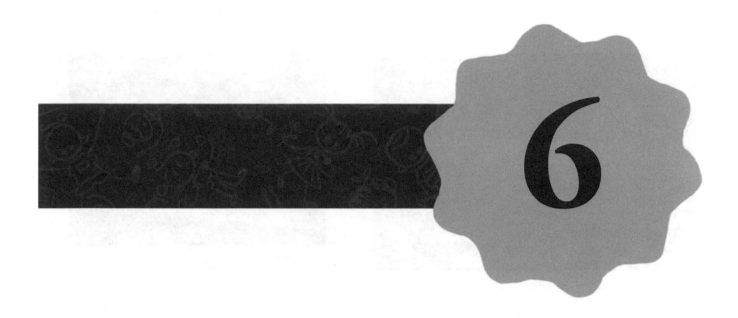

Tactile Sensitivity

Tactile sensitivity and tactile defensiveness are conditions in which a child finds different types of touch aversive. Tactile defensiveness is characterized by a negative response to tactile stimuli (Blakemore et al., 2006). It is postulated that tactile sensitivity may be a result of a lack of habituation in the neural pathways that typically occurs after being exposed repeatedly to a sensory stimulus (Blakemore et al., 2006). A child with tactile sensitivity usually has specific fibers, materials, and foods that are not tolerated (Ayres, 2005). One first must identify these factors before working with the child. Individuals with tactile sensitivity and other sensory defensiveness may be impacted socially, emotionally, and behaviorally (Pfeiffer & Kinnealey, 2003). There is also an increase in "picky eaters" among tactilely defensive children (Nederkoorn et al., 2015).

There are many exercises and activities that can help decrease tactile sensitivity. Some forms of massage have been effective in decreasing tactile sensitivity in children with autism spectrum disorder (Silva & Schalock, 2013). Vibration may also be an effective tool in the treatment of tactile sensitivity (Hochreiter et al., 1983). Firm touch is preferred over light touch and can help suppress sensitivity to light touch (Davich, 2005). In performing the activities in this section, it is important to grade them by presenting the child with the least noxious stimuli and gradually introducing more noxious stimuli. This is done to make sure that the child does not become overly stressed.

ACTIVITIES TO DECREASE TACTILE SENSITIVITY

Deep Pressure

- Lotion massage: Therapist massages child's hands with lotion, applying firm and consistent pressure.
- Squishy toys: Child squeezes and releases toys with different squishy textures.
- Wheelbarrow-walking: Child wheelbarrow-walks across the room.
- While lying prone on a scooter board, child propels self around the room using the palms of their hands.
- Play-Doh: Child plays with Play-Doh, rolling it and squeezing it with both hands.
- Brushing protocol: Refer to Wilbarger's brushing protocol (Wilbarger & Wilbarger, 1991).

Danto, A. H., & Pruzansky, M. *1001 Pediatric Treatment Activities: Creative Ideas for Therapy Sessions, Third Edition* (pp. 41-43).
© 2023 SLACK Incorporated.

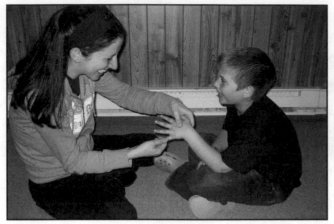

Figure 6-1.

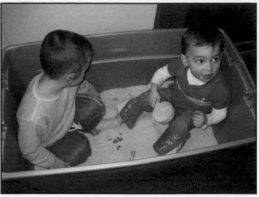

Figure 6-2.

Becoming Comfortable With an Outside Touch

- Graded exposure to textures: Child rubs fabrics of different textures and toys on back and front of the hand as tolerated. Child also attempts this activity with eyes closed and tries to identify objects placed in their hands without the assistance of vision.
- Child strokes the back and front of their hand with a feather.
- Vibrating massage: Child uses a vibrating toy or massager to massage both hands. Child massages both the front and back of the hand as tolerated.
- Vibrating toothbrush: Child brushes teeth with a vibrating toothbrush.
- Therapist plays "This Little Piggy" on the child's fingers (Figure 6-1).
- Face painting: Therapist applies face paint to child's face and cheeks. If child will not tolerate this, allow child to apply the face paint to own face directly.
- Touching faces: Therapist uses fingers to touch different parts of child's face and neck as tolerated. Child labels the body part touched.

Grainy Textures

- Sandbox activities: Child plays in sandbox and makes small castles with sand or finds hidden objects in sand. Additionally, child can make different shapes and letters in the sand.
- Child finds hidden objects in a rice or bean box (Figure 6-2).
- Sandpaper project: Child assists in smoothing rough wood.

Be careful of splinters.

- Child crunches up pieces of corn flakes (or another crunchy cereal) with their hands and sprinkles them onto a piece of paper with glue to make a project.

Creamy and Wet Textures

- Shaving cream activity: Child spreads shaving cream on an inflated balloon. Child then uses their index finger to spell their name in the shaving cream or make a smiley face.
- Finger paint: Child engages in many finger painting projects including making pictures, shapes, and spelling words in the paint.
- Hand-tree project: Therapist places brown paint on child's forearm and hand. Child presses hand onto a white piece of paper. This will provide a tree trunk and branches. Therapist then places different colored paint on child's fingertips and has child press down on the tree branches to make leaves and fruit (Figures 6-3 through 6-5).
- Sticky glue project: Child uses colored or regular glue to squeeze on a piece of paper and then spreads it out with index finger. Child can then place sequins or another craft material on top of the glue.
- Marshmallow Fluff project: Child makes a Marshmallow Fluff sandwich. Child spreads fluff on a piece of bread or cracker with fingers. Allow child to place some toppings onto the fluff (raisins, sprinkles, pretzels, chips, etc.).
- Child spreads peanut butter on a plastic plate—enough to cover the whole surface. Child then spreads chocolate pudding on top of the peanut butter. Child traces different letters on the plate. Allow child to lick finger after each letter.

Be sure to first check for food allergies.

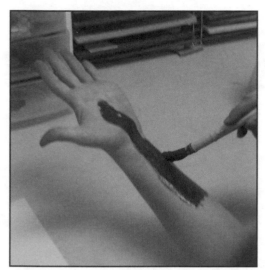

Figure 6-3.

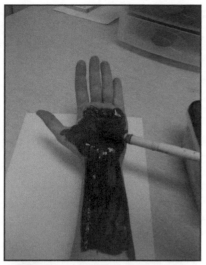

Figure 6-4.

- Water play: Child plays with water in a sink, pouring water from one container to another and then onto their hands. Therapist should vary the temperature of the water from warm to cool. Child should then squeeze washcloths and sponges.

Be sure to supervise this activity to make sure that the water temperature does not become dangerously hot.

- Water hunt: Therapist blindfolds child and asks child to pick out certain objects from the water.

Therapist must use sound judgment in selecting blindfolding activity with a specific child and must carefully supervise any activity involving blindfolding.

- Kneading activities: Child kneads bread or cookie dough to make a baking project.
- Silly Putty: Child pulls Silly Putty and presses it onto different surfaces.
- Play-Doh: Child rolls and pinches Play-Doh.
- Papier-mâché piñata: Child dips strips of newspaper into papier-mâché flour/water mixture and places them on an inflated balloon. Child covers the entire surface except for a small opening at the top. The newspaper is allowed to harden for 1 day then a small opening is cut in the top. Finally the balloon is painted and candy is placed inside.
- Juice making: Child squeezes oranges or grapes into a cup to make fresh juice.

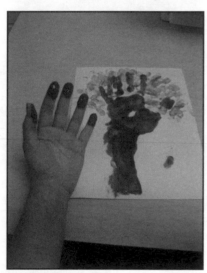

Figure 6-5.

Commercially Available Products

- Playfoam
- Guidecraft 3D Feel & Find Game
- Image Captor
- Kinetic Sand

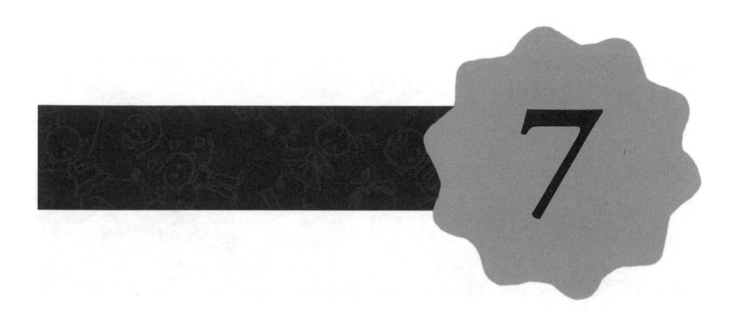

Oral Motor Exercises

Oral motor exercises consist of activities that require the use of the tongue, mouth, lips, and surrounding facial muscles. Many clinicians report seeing a correlation between oral motor exercises and improved motoric abilities and awareness (Muttiah et al., 2011). The purpose of oral motor exercises can be either to strengthen, stimulate, or increase oral motor awareness. Oral motor exercises are most commonly utilized with children with childhood apraxia, low muscle tone, and oral defensiveness (Muttiah et al., 2011). Various oral motor exercises and massages can also be effective with helping children develop adequate oral motor strength and movement for feeding and drinking (Kumin et al., 2001).

These activities and exercises can be performed in preparation for another activity or as an activity in itself. It is important to watch for signs of fatigue when a child is performing these exercises. If the child has feeding/swallowing difficulties, it is important to first check with a doctor or speech therapist before attempting these activities. When working on oral motor issues, the treating therapist should check for the presence of a bite reflex. It is also important to avoid placing small objects in the mouth of a child who may have a tendency to eat nonfood objects.

ORAL MOTOR EXERCISES

Increasing Lip Closure and Cheek Strength

- Child blows bubbles on a bubble wand or bubble stick.
- Child sticks a straw into a cup or bowl filled with water and blows down to create bubbles.
- Child plays with blower toys (Figure 7-1).
- Child blows into whistles and kazoos.
- Therapist teaches child how to play a song on a recorder or asks child to make fun noises with the recorder.
- Child blows pom-poms or cotton balls across a table (Figure 7-2).
- Therapist cuts out a paper fish and places it on a table. Child then blows it into a specific target (e.g., into a bucket with water).
- Therapist tapes a small piece of paper or a feather to the end of a straw and asks the child to blow through the straw (Figure 7-3).

Danto, A. H., & Pruzansky, M. *1001 Pediatric Treatment Activities:*
Creative Ideas for Therapy Sessions, Third Edition (pp. 45-48).
© 2023 SLACK Incorporated.

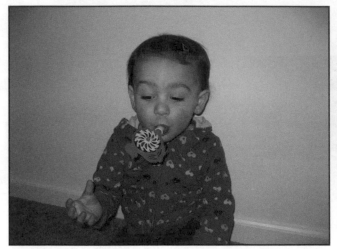

Figure 7-1.

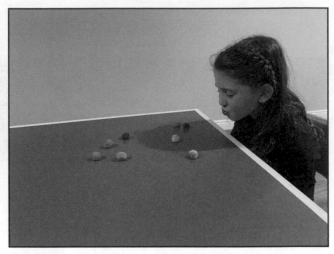

Figure 7-2.

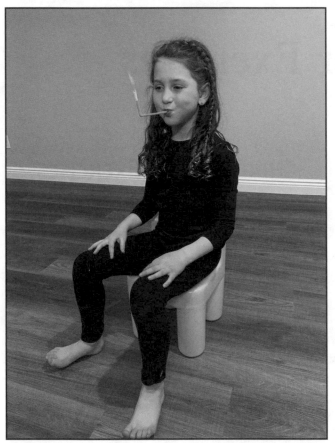

Figure 7-3.

Sound Making

Therapist makes different sounds and noises and attempts to get child to imitate them.

Therapist and child sing a song with many different sounds. For example, sing "Witch Doctor" ("Ooo eee ooo ah ah") or "Old McDonald Had a Farm" ("Ee i ee i oh") to practice making different sounds in a fun way.

Exercises for Overall Strengthening of Oral Structures

Therapist should first check for any dental problems the child may have or for issues with bite reflexes.

- Jaw-strengthening exercises: Child bites down on Popsicle stick while therapist pulls on it, or child places a Popsicle stick horizontally in mouth and bites down using teeth (Figures 7-4 and 7-5).

- Lip-strengthening exercises: Therapist places a Popsicle stick between child's lips and has child hold this position (Figure 7-6).

- Tongue tug-of-war: Therapist wraps gauze around child's tongue and gently pulls it out of child's mouth. The child is asked to try to resist.

- Cheek thrusts: Child pushes tongue into the side of the mouth to make one cheek stick out. Therapist pushes against the side of child's cheek, trying to push against the tongue.

- Tongue push-ups: Child places a Cheerio, M&M's, or a Froot Loop on top of the tongue and pushes tongue up against the palate for a couple seconds at a time, gradually increasing the amount of time the tongue can stay pushed to the top of the mouth.

- Gum chewing: Therapist places gum on the child's back molars and asks child to practice biting up and down, gradually increasing amount of times they can bite down (Rosenfeld-Johnson, 2001, pp. 110-117 [Review Rosenfeld-Johnson reference for sample gum-chewing protocol.]).

- Child sucks liquids through a crazy straw. Therapist should vary the thickness and texture of the liquids.

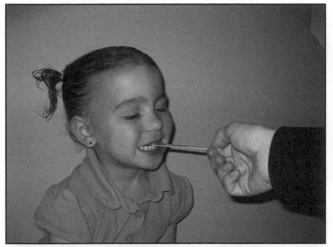

Figure 7-4.

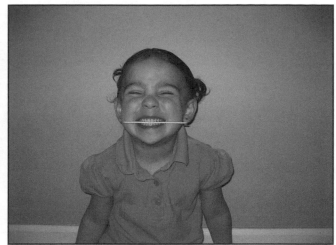

Figure 7-5.

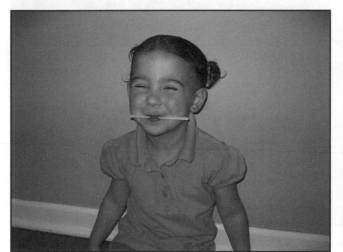

Figure 7-6.

- Therapist places jelly/Marshmallow Fluff/peanut butter on the roof of child's mouth and has child lick it off.
- Therapist places jelly/Marshmallow Fluff/peanut butter on the top lip and has child lick it off (Figure 7-7).
- Therapist provides child with crunchy and sticky foods to chew.
- Child copies tongue movements and positions, including up, down, side to side, and all around.
- Child copies lip positions, including purse, pucker, smile, frown, open, and close.
- Tongue scavenger hunt: Therapist touches child's lips and the skin around the mouth or any spot inside the mouth with either a tongue depressor or a lollipop. Child then must point to the spot touched with the tip of the tongue.
- Fish face: Child tries to imitate a "fish face," holds the position for several seconds, and then relaxes the facial muscles. Repeat as tolerated (Figure 7-8).

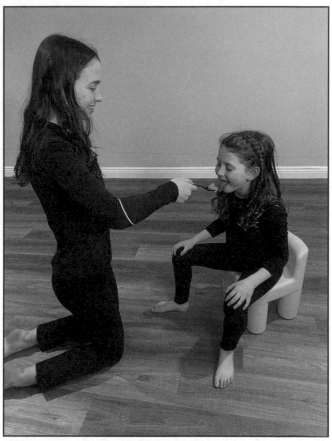

Figure 7-7.

- Therapist places a small amount of ChapStick on the child's lips and has child try to spread the ChapStick onto the entire surface of the lips by closing their lips together and moving them back and forth, without using the hands.

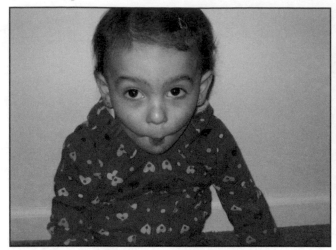

Figure 7-8.

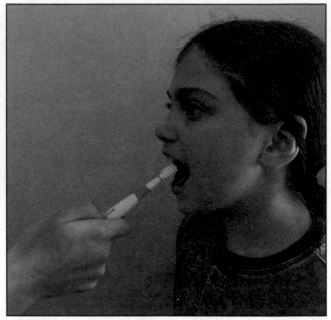

Figure 7-9.

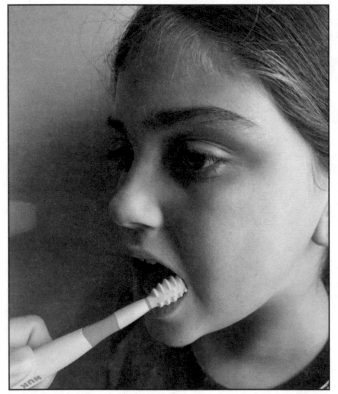

Figure 7-10.

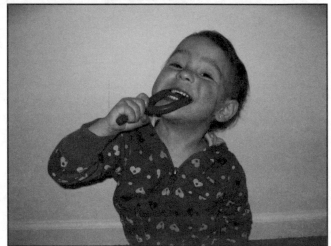

Figure 7-11.

Stimulating the Mouth Through Sensory Input

- Therapist provides compression with fingers to child's back molars. (Therapist should be wearing gloves. Check first for latex allergies.)
- Therapist touches and massages different parts of child's face with a warm and cold wet cloth.

- Therapist gently taps the skin with fingers around the child's mouth and has the child do the same.
- Child places Z-Vibe toy in mouth to gently stimulate different parts of the mouth (lips, tongue, cheeks) with vibration and rubbing.
- Therapist stimulates different areas in and around the mouth with a Nuk Brush (Figures 7-9 and 7-10).
- Therapist massages different parts of child's face and surrounding area with lotion.
- Plain facial and lip massage: Therapist gently massages the skin around the child's mouth and the lips as tolerated.
- ARK's Grabbers/Chewy Tubes: Child bites down and releases on chewy toy (Figure 7-11).

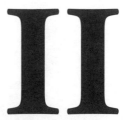

Visual System

Many consider the visual system to be the most dominant and influential system in the human body (Schneck, 1996). The body uses the visual system to obtain information about the environment. Dysfunction in the visual system can negatively affect quality of life and decrease functional independence with activities of daily living (Markowitz, 2006).

This section focuses on three main components of the visual system: visual perception, visual motor integration, and oculomotor movement.

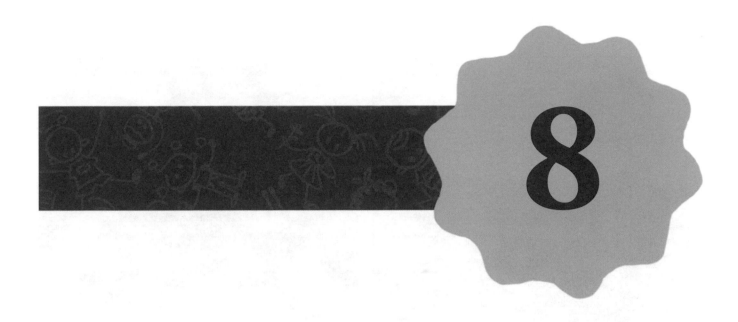

Visual Perception

Visual perception involves the process of receiving information from the environment and translating the input into meaning (Cooke et al., 2005). Visual perception has seven main components: visual discrimination (the ability to discriminate between two similar forms), visual form constancy (the ability to recognize the same form when it appears in a different way), visual figure/ground (the ability to find a form when it is hidden among other forms), visual closure (the ability to recognize a form when the complete form is not visible), visual spatial relations (the ability to determine the correct direction of forms), visual memory (the ability to remember the details of a single form), and visual sequential memory (the ability to remember and recall a sequence of objects; Martin, 2006).

Impairments with visual perceptual skills may cause difficulties processing, organizing, and interpreting visual information the brain receives (Cooke et al., 2005). In one survey of Australian occupational therapists regarding which performance components they evaluate in children with learning disabilities, 100% of respondents indicated visual perceptual skills (Wallen & Walker, 1995). Visual perceptual deficits can also impair reading and writing tasks as well (Cooke et al., 2005). Visual perceptual skills are a commonly targeted area by pediatric occupational therapists (Schneck, 1996).

This chapter provides a variety of visual perceptual exercises that can help strengthen the visual perceptual system through fun games and activities.

VISUAL PERCEPTUAL ACTIVITIES

Visual Discrimination

- Child completes "What's Missing/What's Different Pictures." (See Appendix A, pp. 203-204, for sample pictures.)

- Therapist shows child a string of four different pictures and asks child to figure out which two pictures are exactly alike and circle them. (See Appendix A, pp. 205-207, for sample pictures.)

- Dot marker game: Using different colored markers, the therapist makes circles of various colors and sizes on a page. Child should then be given dot markers and be told to place the corresponding colored dot into each circle on the page (Figure 8-1). (See Appendix A, p. 208, for sample dot marker handout.)

Danto, A. H., & Pruzansky, M. *1001 Pediatric Treatment Activities: Creative Ideas for Therapy Sessions, Third Edition* (pp. 51-56).
© 2023 SLACK Incorporated.

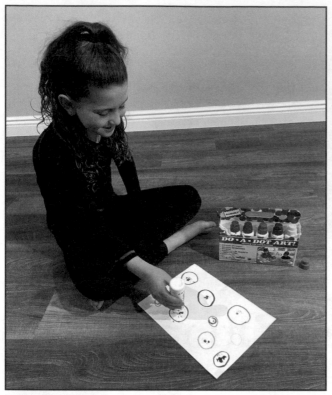

Figure 8-1.

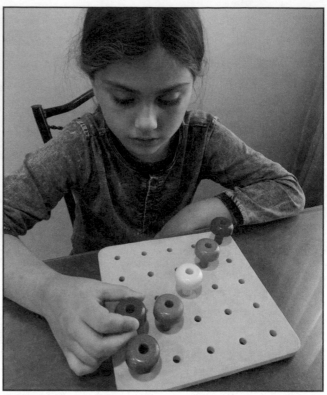

Figure 8-2.

- Verbal descriptions: In learning how to write new letters, therapist has child verbally describe the letter. This may help the child remember the different attributes of a letter and be able to write and recognize it more easily.
- Sorting games
  - Puzzle piece sorting: Child assists in sorting center puzzle pieces from edge puzzle pieces.
  - Child plays with color and shape sorters.
  - Baseball or any sport card sorting: Child sorts players by team, league, etc.
  - Deck of cards: Child sorts cards by suit, number, etc.
  - Froot Loops sorting activity: Therapist places Froot Loops all over table and gives child five strings. Child makes five different necklaces that are all one specific color.
- Copying patterns
  - Froot Loops necklaces: Therapist places different colored Froot Loops on a string to make a necklace. Child copies the pattern of colors on the original necklace. This activity can be upgraded or downgraded based on the complexity of the pattern and the number of colors used in making the necklace (i.e., use anywhere from two to six colors when creating the original pattern).
  - Peg patterns: Child places pegs into a peg board in a specific order, copying a set pattern made by the therapist (Figure 8-2).

  - Necklace making: Therapist provides child with different colored beads and has child copy a pattern with the beads.

Visual Form Constancy

- Ball-bouncing game
  - Part I: Therapist places different random letters on the wall and asks child to spell a word by throwing a ball against the letters, one at a time and in the correct order, to spell the word.
  - Part II: Child covers eyes while therapist flips the letters on the wall so the letters are upside down, sideways, or backward. Child opens eyes to look at the letters and tries and spell the same word.
- Letter recognition: Therapist writes the letters of the alphabet in different ways on multiple index cards or pieces of paper. For example therapist can write the letter "A" in a big size, little size, uppercase, lowercase, cursive, red, blue, and yellow. Therapist should do this for several more letters, mix the letters up, and scatter them on the floor. Child should then try and find all of the different As hidden on the floor and subsequently the other letters as well.
- View Appendix A, pp. 209-210, for form constancy handout.

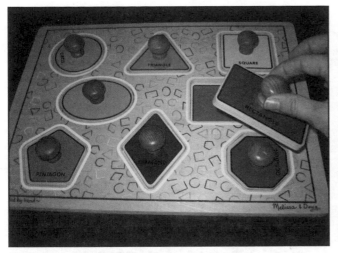

Figure 8-3.

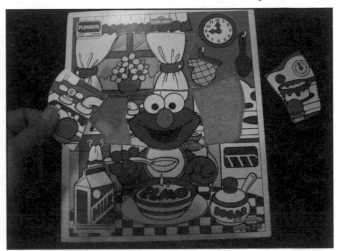

Figure 8-4.

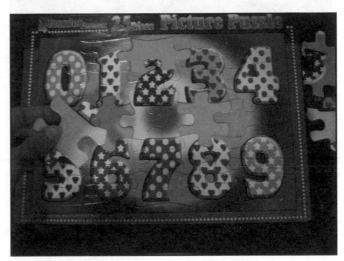

Figure 8-5.

Visual Figure/Ground

- Compensatory strategies to help a child with poor figure ground skills include the following:
  - Limit visual distractions by keeping a child's work area free of clutter.
  - Have child sit in the front of the classroom to limit visual distractions.
  - When providing a written assignment for the child, write as little on every page as possible. For example, for a math homework assignment, write only one math problem on each page.
  - Use bright, colorful borders around the paper the child is writing on to give an additional visual cue. Some children might find this distracting and may benefit more from a dark black border around the paper they are working on.
- Hidden pictures: Child finds different hidden objects in a picture. (See Appendix A, pp. 211-212, for sample hidden picture handout.)
- Child completes word searches/word finds.
- Finding objects in a competing background: Child finds a specific toy either somewhere in the room or on a messy shelf among other toys.
- Therapist places laminated letters all around floor and has child jump over, hop over, or touch the letters of child's name.
- I Spy: Therapist should look around the room and think of an object in the room. Therapist should give clues about the object (e.g., size, color, specific features). Child has to look around the room to find it. Child is allowed to ask for hints and other clues.

- Find the Letter: Child copies a word, sentence, or paragraph onto a piece of paper. Therapist provides child with a red pen or marker. Child then goes back to composition and looks for a specific letter. For example, choose the letter "R." Have the child read over the written work and circle all of the Rs on the page.

Visual Closure

- Puzzles: Child completes different puzzles.
  - The easiest type of puzzle is a form puzzle (Figure 8-3).
  - The next level of difficulty is a cut puzzle (Figure 8-4).
  - The most challenging type of puzzle is an interlocking puzzle (Figure 8-5).

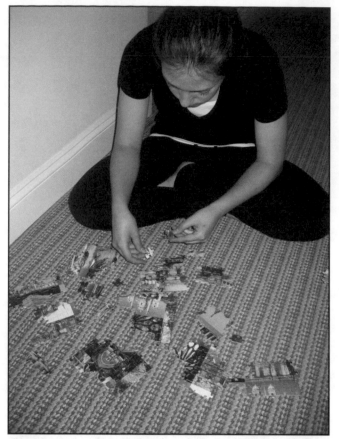

Figure 8-6.

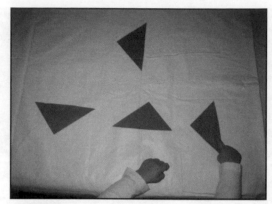

Figure 8-7.

- Child completes interlocking puzzle with many small pieces (Figure 8-6).

- When putting a puzzle together, therapist asks child to identify an object in a specific puzzle piece without looking at the completed puzzle picture.

- Incomplete puzzles: Therapist assists child in putting together a puzzle, but hides several pieces of the puzzle. Therapist asks child to identify what is the picture in the puzzle with only part of the puzzle completed.

- Letter identification: Therapist writes parts of a letter on a paper and asks child to identify which letter it is. (See Appendix A, p. 213, for sample handout.)

- Word identification: Therapist writes parts of the different letters in a word to see if the child is able to identify the word. This activity can also be played by covering the bottom quarter of a word with a piece of paper to see if the child can guess the word with only the top three-quarters of the word visible. (See Appendix A, p. 214, for sample handout.)

- Picture identification: Therapist creates a picture and covers up part of it to see if child is able to identify the item in the picture (See Appendix A, pp. 215-216, for sample handout.)

Visual Spatial Relations

- Child completes shape/size sorter worksheet (See Appendix A, pp. 193-196, for handout.)

- Puzzles: Child assists in turning the puzzle pieces in the correct direction.

- Shape matching: Therapist cuts out four items of same shape or picture. Therapist places the shapes on the table with one shape placed on the table above the other three. The three shapes should all be facing a different direction with only one of them placed in the same direction as the shape on top of the others. Child then identifies which shape matches the direction of the shape on top (Figure 8-7).

- LEGO matching: This game is the same as the shape matching game (listed earlier), but played with LEGO pieces. Therapist places four of the exact same LEGO pieces on the table. One of the LEGO pieces should be in a row of its own on top of the other three. The bottom three LEGO pieces should all face a different direction from each other, except one should face the same direction as the LEGO piece on top. Child picks which LEGO piece is facing the same direction as the one on top.

- Keyholes: Therapist draws a picture of a pretend keyhole and picture of a pretend key. Therapist cuts out the key and asks child to turn the key in the correct direction needed to place the key into the hole.

- SET: Child plays the commercially available card game of SET with another child in order to find shapes/patterns with different orientations and colors (Figure 8-8).

- Oops letter writing: Therapist deliberately writes a letter on the board with an error (upside down, backward, etc.). Child tries to verbally describe the error with the letter.

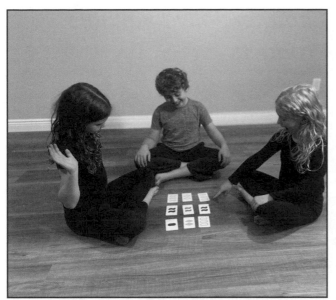

Figure 8-8.

- Be the teacher: Child copies a sentence or writes a composition on a piece of lined paper. Provide the child with a special felt-tipped marker or pen. Have the child go back and edit the paper, circling every letter that does not properly reach the line or letters that erroneously go below the line. Give the child one point for every correct circle and ask the child to try to reach a set score.

- A child who has difficulty writing neatly in a confined space may be having difficulty with visual spatial relations. It may be helpful to use different types of paper in order to help a child visualize the correct place on the paper to write. Such papers include the following:

  ○ Graph paper: Child writes one letter per each slot on the graph paper (Figures 8-9 and 8-10). Use smaller or bigger boxed graph paper based on the child's handwriting level. The smaller the boxes, the more difficult the handwriting activity is.

  ○ Raised line paper: This type of paper can help a child feel a physical boundary when writing.

  ○ Visual clues: Therapist colors over the margin line with a thick red marker to remind the child the starting place to come back to when they finish writing on a specific line. Therapist can also highlight parts of the paper.

  ○ Additional visual cues: A child who has difficulty organizing overall writing may require some other visual cue aside from the margin line. It may be helpful to place a sticker or a star in the upper left corner of the page to remind the child where writing starts. Handwriting Without Tears provides prefabricated paper like this.

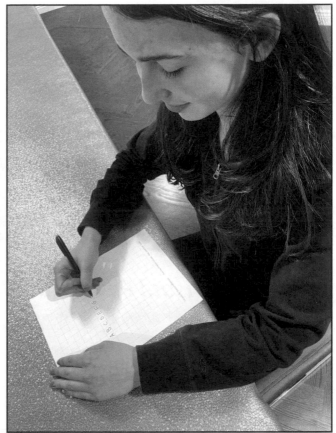

Figure 8-9.

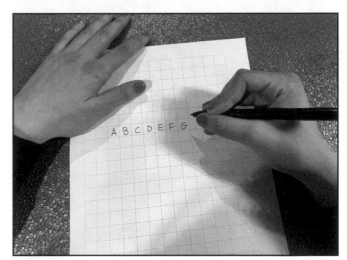

Figure 8-10.

Visual Memory

- Memory games: These can be played with an actual Memory game or can be self-made. Therapist places pairs of cards face down on the table. Child flips over two cards each turn, trying to find a match.

- Froot Loops Memory game: Therapist shows the child a card with a sequence of colors written on it—for example: red, orange, yellow, blue. The card is then removed and the child makes a Froot Loops necklace with the correct order of colors.

- "Busy picture" books: Child looks at a page on a "busy picture" book for a little while. The book is then closed and the child tells the therapist as many details about the page as possible.

Additional Visual Perceptual Resources

- *Test of Visual Perceptual Skills, Revised* (TVPS-R). The TVPS-R is meant to be used as an evaluation tool to test a child's visual perceptual skills. The TVPS-R offers many examples of visual perception challenges. A therapist can look at the items in this evaluation in order to see various examples of visual perception challenges and create new ones based off these samples.

Online

Visit the following website for additional visual perceptual activities: http://edhelper.com/visual_skills.htm

Commercially Available Products

- Colorama
- Connect Four
- Design and Drill Activity Center
- Dominoes
- Doodle Dice Deluxe
- Fantacolor Junior
- I Spy
- Katamino
- KID K'NEX
- Lincoln Logs
- Oreo Matchin' Middle
- Pattern Blocks & Board
- Pattern Play
- Perfection
- Picture Perfect Design Tiles
- Rainbow Loom
- Rush Hour Jr.
- SET
- Smart Snacks Mix & Match Doughnut
- Smart Snacks Sorting Shapes Cupcakes
- Spot It
- Stare!
- Tetris
- Tic-Tac-Toe
- Where's Waldo

9

Visual Motor Integration

Visual motor integration (VMI) refers to the coordination of visual perception and the movement of the fingers (Beery, 2004). Visual motor skills have been found to be correlated with school readiness, school adjustment, and social-emotional well being (Bart et al., 2007). VMI skills affect a child's ability to cut with scissors, complete mazes, stack blocks, and be successful in most sport activities. Decreased visual motor skills can be related to clumsiness in children as well (Parush et al., 1998). VMI is also a required skill necessary for handwriting legibility (Daly et al., 2003)

When working on visual motor skills, there are aspects of VMI that can pose difficulties for the child (i.e., the motor component, the perceptual component, or both can be equally troublesome). For example, a child who has difficulty completing mazes may struggle with moving a pencil through the maze within a confined space, but may easily be able to see the correct path with their eyes. Conversely, another child may be able to guide a pencil through the same maze with no problem, but have difficulty locating the correct path visually. Therefore, in selecting visual motor exercises, it is important to identify which component of VMI is difficult for the particular child.

This chapter provides a variety of VMI activities. It is important to remember that VMI activities call upon both perceptual and motor skills; one must keep this in mind when determining an appropriate choice of activity to challenge the child.

VISUAL MOTOR ACTIVITIES

Cutting and Gluing

- Cutting practice
  - Child snips a narrow sheet of paper (Figure 9-1).
  - Child cuts on straight lines.
  - Child cuts out shapes. (See Appendix A, pp. 193-196, for shape cutouts.)
  - Child cuts out pictures.
- Cutting textures: Child cuts out paper, cardboard, straw, Play-Doh, and Silly Putty.
- Child squeezes glue onto a line.

Danto, A. H., & Pruzansky, M. *1001 Pediatric Treatment Activities: Creative Ideas for Therapy Sessions, Third Edition* (pp. 57-62).
© 2023 SLACK Incorporated.

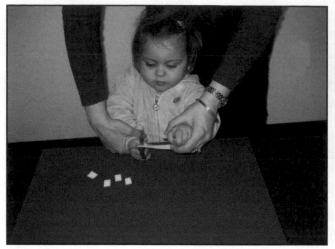

Figure 9-1.

Handwriting Skills Involving Writing/Drawing

- Child completes dot-to-dots. (See Appendix A, pp. 217-221, for sample dot-to-dots.)

- Child completes mazes. (See Appendix A, pp. 222-226, for varying level mazes.)

- Child traces between lines or along shapes or pictures. (See Appendix A, pp. 197-202 and 227-233, for tracing handouts.)

- Handprint making: Child places nondominant hand on a piece of paper and uses the dominant hand to trace out the hand on the paper.

- Child completes follow the arrow handout (see Appendix A, p. 234, for sample handout).

- Cage the animal: Therapist draws a picture of any animal inside a box. Therapist tells child that the animal will escape if bars are not drawn onto the animal's cage. Child draws straight lines from the top of the cage to the bottom of the cage.

- Copying lines, prewriting strokes, and shapes: Child copies different simple shapes, letters, words, sentences, or paragraphs onto a piece of paper.

- Copying images: Child copies a series of different complex figures and drawings. Keep in mind appropriate age expectations when having a child complete this activity. A child should not be asked to copy a figure that is developmentally too sophisticated. See the *Beery Developmental Test of Visual Motor Integration* as a resource for age appropriate expectations (Beery et al., 2010).

- Child uses stencils to make drawings and pictures.

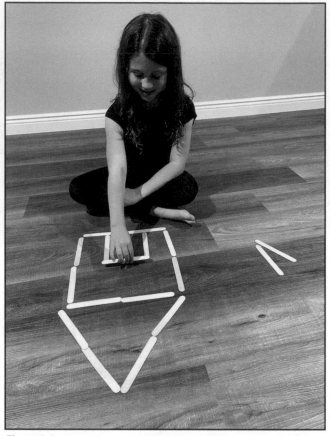

Figure 9-2.

Building

- Child builds a house with Popsicle sticks (Figure 9-2).

- Create a box with Popsicle sticks: Therapist overlaps sticks on different layers and then has child copy the template design (Figure 9-3).

- Building/stacking: Child builds and stacks blocks and cubes to make a tower.

- Therapist creates a small design or tower with blocks or cubes and has child try to replicate the design or tower.

- Marshmallow building: Therapist creates different geometrical designs using marshmallows with toothpicks connecting the shape together. Child copies designs (Figure 9-4).

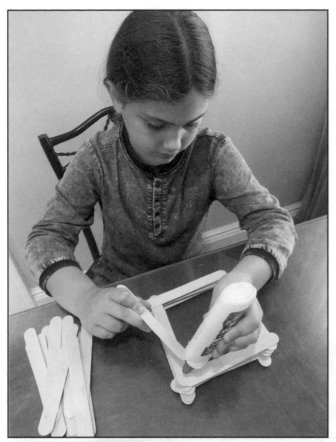

Figure 9-3.

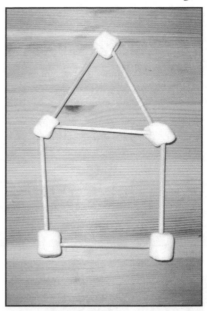

Figure 9-4.

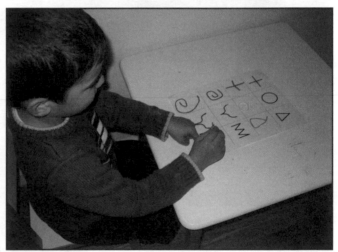

Figure 9-6.

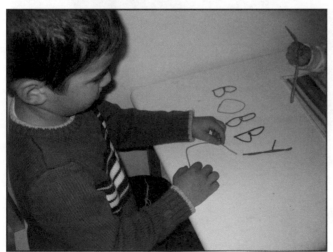

Figure 9-5.

Forming Letters, Shapes, and Designs

- Pipe cleaner letters: Child copies models of letters with pipe cleaners and then creates letters independently with a pipe cleaner (without a model to look at).

- Play-Doh letters: Child copies letters with Play-Doh and then creates letters independently with Play-Doh (without a model to look at).

- Therapist gives out Popsicle sticks. Child makes shapes and letters with Popsicle sticks.

- Child makes letters with Wikki Stix (Figure 9-5).

- Child copies designs and patterns with Wikki Stix (Figures 9-6 and 9-7; see sample handout in Appendix A, p. 235, of designs child can copy with Wikki Stix.)

- Therapist cuts out pieces of string or colored lanyard of different lengths and places the pieces in random patterns, overlapping them. Child tries to place strings in the same design as in the template (Figure 9-8).

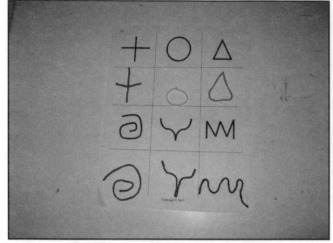

Figure 9-7.

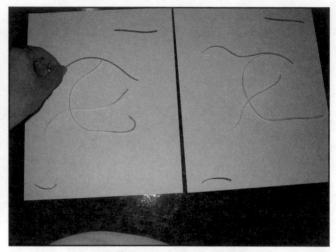

Figure 9-8.

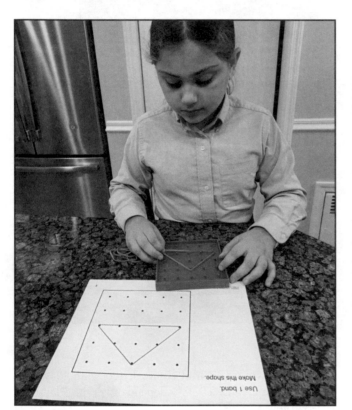

Figure 9-9.

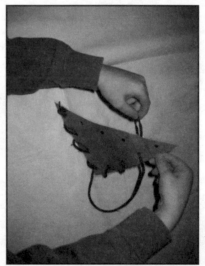

Figure 9-10.

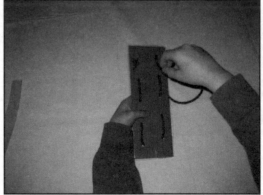

Figure 9-11.

- Geoboards: Child copies designs and shapes on a geoboard (Figure 9-9).
- Lacing boards: Child uses a lacing board and practices going around the lacing board with a whip stitch (Figure 9-10) and then an over-under stitch (Figure 9-11).

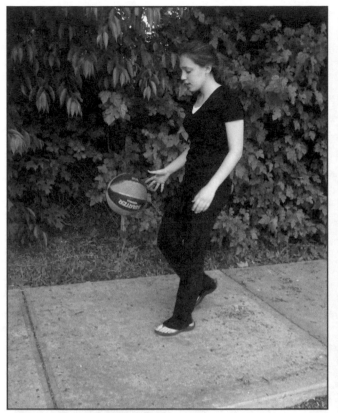

Figure 9-12.

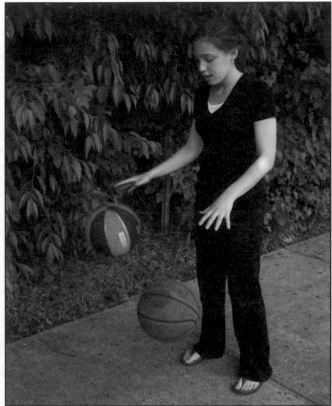

Figure 9-13.

Ball Games

- Dribbling activities
  - ○ Child practices dribbling a basketball quickly and slowly (Figure 9-12).
  - ○ Child practices dribbling a ball with each hand simultaneously (Figure 9-13).
- HORSE: Child plays the basketball game HORSE with another child or therapist. Child shoots a ball in a basketball hoop. If the child misses the shot, it is the therapist's turn. If the child makes the shot, the therapist must make the same shot. If the therapist misses, they get a letter of the word "HORSE." If the therapist makes the shot, it is then the child's turn again to shoot a different shot, and so on. Whoever gets all letters and spells HORSE loses the game.
- Bowling: Therapist sets up bowling pins or soft blocks. Child bowls with a small- or medium-sized ball and tries to knock over as many pins/blocks as possible.
- Juggling
  - ○ Therapist teaches child how to juggle three or more balls (Figure 9-14).

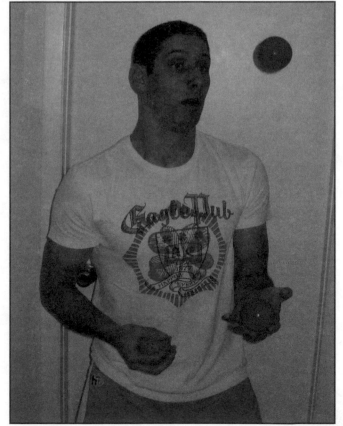

Figure 9-14.

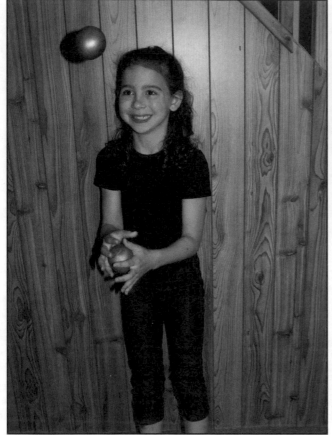

Figure 9-15.

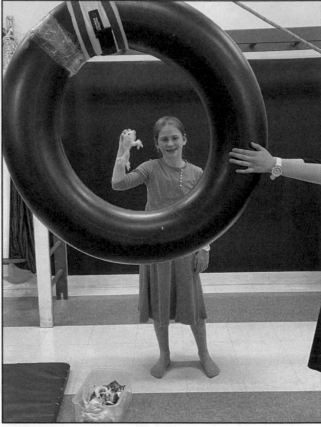

Figure 9-16.

○ Child holds two balls, one ball in each hand. Child throws right ball up and then passes ball from left hand to right hand and catches the ball in the air with left hand. Repeat activity multiple times (Figure 9-15).

• Tic-tock-tire: Therapist hangs up a suspended tire swing (or a Hula Hoop) and swings it from side to side. Therapist places a bucket full of small items (bean bags, Koosh balls, etc.) on the floor to the side of the child. Child picks up one item at a time and throws it through the moving tire without letting the bean bags touch the tire (Figure 9-16).

Folding Activities

• Origami: Therapist creates simple origami designs for child to copy.

• Paper airplanes: Therapist creates a paper airplane and has child copy the steps, one step at a time.

• Dinner napkin folding: Therapist teaches child simple ways to fold dinner napkins. Different fun ideas can be found online by searching for "easy napkin folding."

Online

• Visit www.eyecanlearn.com for additional visual motor activities that can be played on a computer.

Commercially Available Products

• Angry Birds Mega Smash

• Elefun

• Frisbee

• Jacks

• Labyrinth

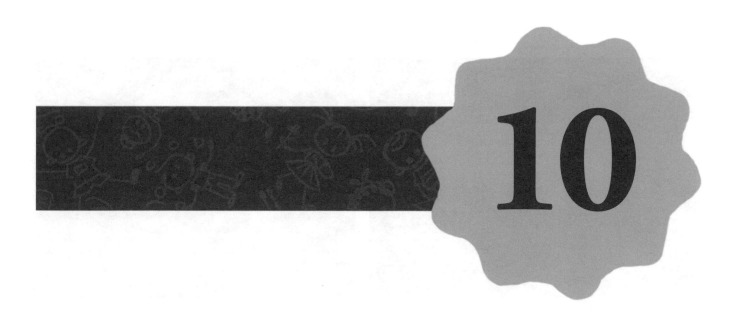

Oculomotor Exercises

The four major components of the oculomotor system include saccadic movements, smooth pursuits, convergence, and the vestibular system (Robinson, 1968). Although oculomotor movement can be a broad term that encompasses many different areas, this section focuses on a few specific components. These include tracking a slow-moving object, moving the eyes quickly between two close objects, and moving the eyes from an object that is close to an object that is far away.

Decreased oculomotor movement may affect both academic and functional skills. Different abilities of the visual system are highly correlated to a child's success with reading skills and overall academic performance (Kavale, 1982). Functionally, a child may have difficulty playing sports and simply being able to watch moving objects in the environment.

Children with poor visual scanning skills will often compensate for this deficit by moving their heads instead of using isolated eye movements when tracking something. This results in inefficient and ineffective visual scanning. It is important with vision exercises to keep the head still (Axelsson et al., 2019). It may also be necessary for the treating therapist to provide gentle physical input to serve as a reminder to keep the head still during the exercises. If the head moves when these exercises are performed, the child will not be improving their oculomotor abilities to the optimal level.

This chapter provides many oculomotor exercises. Included is a group of exercises that call for visual scanning activities involving balance. These exercises are incorporated into this chapter because a child exists in a dynamic environment. Sensory information from both the visual and vestibular system share brain-way pathway connections and help produce motor output that affects body posture and balance (Jones et al., 2009). Children must learn to scan on static surfaces as well as dynamic ones. For example, a child might want to read a street sign while walking on a bumpy sidewalk, ascending a flight of stairs, or stepping up onto a curb.

As the visual system has a strong connection to the system controlling movement, a therapist must watch for signs of dizziness when performing oculomotor exercises and stop immediately if a child reports being either dizzy or nauseous.

Danto, A. H., & Pruzansky, M. *1001 Pediatric Treatment Activities: Creative Ideas for Therapy Sessions, Third Edition* (pp. 63-70).
© 2023 SLACK Incorporated.

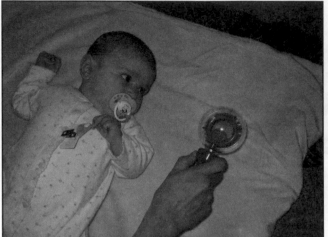

Figure 10-1.

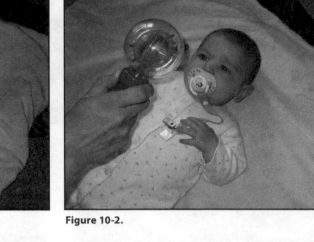

Figure 10-2.

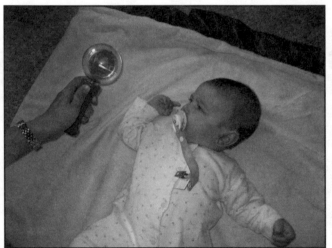

Figure 10-3.

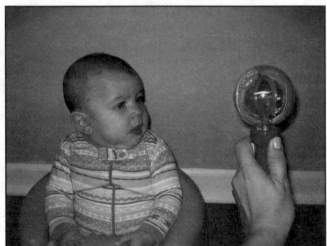

Figure 10-4.

Visual Scanning Activities

Basic Visual Tracking

To increase isolated eye movements instead of full head movements, it might be helpful to lightly hold the child's head still, forcing the child to move the eyes only and not the head.

- Visual tracking for the higher-level child: Therapist holds an object in front of child's face. Therapist instructs child to look at the moving object with only their eyes and not to move the head. Therapist should alternate moving the object slowly and quickly in all different planes. Therapist should try to pick something visually attractive in order to help the child maintain visual attention (e.g., finger puppet, toy with lights).

- Visual tracking for lower-level child or young child (to be determined by therapist): Place child in upright, seated position or flat on back. Move a toy/object of interest/shining light around child. Move the toy or light in an arc from side to side, up and down, and in both diagonal planes.

  ○ On back (Figures 10-1 through 10-3).

  ○ Sitting upright (Figures 10-4 through 10-6).

- Practicing saccades (i.e., the ability to quickly move the eyes from one target to another): Therapist holds up one object in each hand and asks child to look at each object alternately in a random pattern. For example, therapist can hold a red marble and a blue marble. Therapist then calls out "red, blue, red, blue," etc. Therapist moves the two objects around/up/down, while child looks back and forth between them, keeping the head still (Figure 10-7). Therapist should alternate timing between verbal cues to decrease habit/patterning.

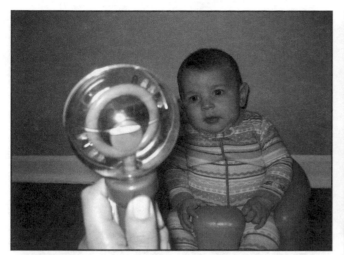

Figure 10-5.

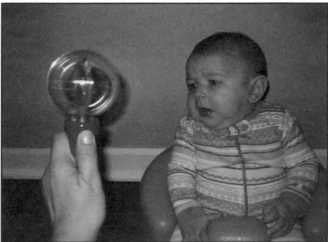

Figure 10-6.

- Flashlight tag: This game should be played in a dark room. Therapist shines a light on the ceiling or somewhere else in the room. Child quickly locates this light and shines a flashlight next to it.

- "Where is it": Therapist places a penny or small object on the table in front of child. Therapist picks it up with one hand and transfers it back and forth between hands several times as the child watches. When the therapist stops, child must guess which hand is holding the penny.

- Reading exercises

  ○ Child holds book in hand and reads out loud to therapist.

  ○ Child reads book, keeping the index finger under the word being read.

  ○ Child reads a row of letters placed on the board X feet away (appropriate distance should be determined by treating therapist).

  ○ Child reads a list of sentences placed on the wall X feet away (appropriate distance should be determined by treating therapist).

- "Where is the queen": Therapist places three playing cards face up on the table. One of the cards should be a queen. Therapist shows the child where the queen is and then turns the cards face down. Therapist slowly moves the cards around; then the child has to point to the card that they believe is the queen card.

- Bead mazes: Child pushes the beads from one side of the bead maze to the other (Figure 10-8).

- Yo-yo activities: Therapist has child watch yo-yo as it is moved up and down and then swung gently from side to side. Therapist instructs child of appropriate age to attempt swinging yo-yo (this will be too difficult for younger children).

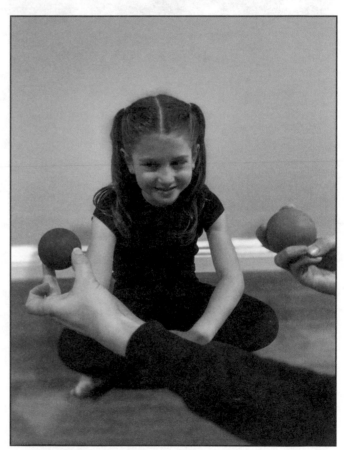

Figure 10-7.

Visual Scanning Activities Involving Balance

- Balance beam scanning game: Child walks across a balance beam while reading across a row on a letter chart placed on the wall at the child's front or side. To upgrade this activity, have child read down a column, read the first and last letters of a row, read every

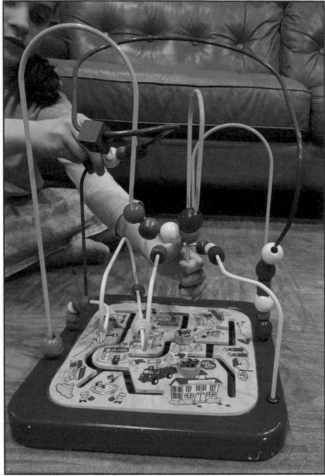

Figure 10-8.

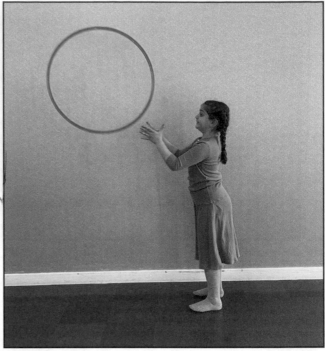

Figure 10-9.

other letter in a row, or read two letters at a time. This activity can be made simpler by placing a long strip of masking tape on the floor and having the child walk across the masking tape instead of the balance beam when reading the letters. If a child does not yet know the names of the letters, an alternative picture/symbol chart can be used. (See Appendix A, pp. 236-237, for letter and symbol chart.)

- Slow movement tips: Child sits in a chair facing therapist. Therapist holds child's head and maintains eye contact with child. Therapist slowly moves child's head in different directions, including right, left, backward, and forward.

- Heel-toe rocking: Child maintains balance on heels. They then rock back and forth between heels and toes, holding each position for approximately 1 to 2 seconds. Once child is able to perform this activity smoothly, therapist places a sentence on the wall that the child must read while rocking back and forth between heels and toes.

Writing/Drawing

- Matching cars games: Therapist takes a piece of paper and on the far right side of the page makes a column with different cars and on the far left side of the page writes different numbers. Draw lines between the cars and numbers and ask the child to use only their eyes to see where each vehicle ended up. (See Appendix A, pp. 238-240, for sample handouts.)

- Copying words and sentences: Child copies words or sentences from a blackboard onto a paper placed on a table or desk in front of the child.

- Copying words and sentences: Child copies words or sentences out of a book placed on the table directly in front of the child.

- Blowing bubbles: Child stands on floor or on a balance beam. Therapist blows bubbles all around child. Child tries to pop as many bubbles as possible.

Throw/Catch and Ball Activities

- Child throws a Hula Hoop in the air and catches it (Figure 10-9).

- Hula Hoop toss: Child and therapist both hold a Hula Hoop in their hands. When therapist calls out "go," they each throw their Hula Hoop and catch the other person's Hula Hoop simultaneously (Figure 10-10).

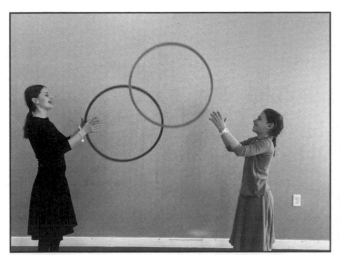

Figure 10-10.

- ABC wall game: Therapist places the letters "A" through "E" on the wall approximately half an inch apart in a random order. The letters should be large enough so a child can stand a few feet away from the wall and still see them. Child throws a ball at letter "A" and catches ball as it bounces off wall. Child then continues throwing the ball in ABC order and catches it. Therapist can upgrade this activity by adding more letters or downgrade the activity by placing only two or three letters on the wall.

- Wall spelling game: Therapist places scattered letters on the wall in a random order. Therapist calls out a letter and child throws a ball against the corresponding letter and catches it. For older children, therapist calls out a word and child throws the ball at each letter in the word (in the correct order).

- Child plays a sports game that requires a quick-moving ball. Some of these activities include floor hockey, air hockey, miniature golf, Ping-Pong, Frisbee, soccer, hitting a baseball in the air, tennis, etc. (Figure 10-11).

- Balloon air-bouncing: Child hits a balloon with either a racquet or own hand. Child tries to keep the balloon from falling to the floor.

- Balloon volleyball: Child hits a balloon with either a racquet or own hand while playing a game of volleyball with another person.

- Child bounces a small ball between a tennis racket and the floor.

- Child bounces a small ball on top of a tennis racket and keeps it in the air.

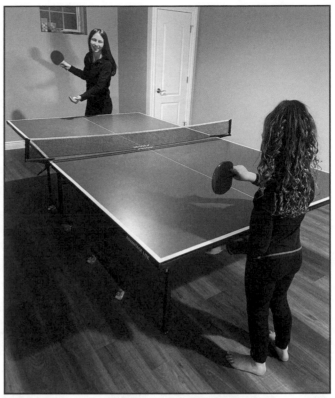

Figure 10-11.

Jumping

- Trampoline letter game: Therapist tapes different letters onto a trampoline. Therapist calls out one letter at a time and child quickly finds the letter and jumps onto it.

- Arrow map: Therapist places arrow map on the wall. (See Appendix A, p. 241, for sample chart.) Child reads the directions of the arrows out loud, walks in the direction of the arrows, jumps in the direction of the arrows, or dances to a beat while moving in the direction of the arrows.

Strengthening Eye Convergence

- Therapist places a small sticker on the wall. Child does wall push-ups while maintaining eye contact on the sticker and has nose touch the sticker each time the body is brought in close to the wall (Figure 10-12).

- Suspended ball activities: Child hits a suspended ball or tether ball with hand or any sort of rod. Upgrade the activity by taping colored lines on a rod and have child only hit the ball with a specific color. Further upgrade this activity by performing it on a balance board (Figure 10-13).

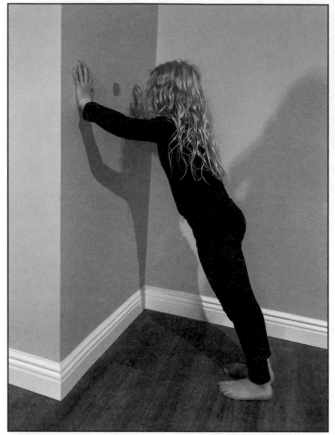

Figure 10-12.

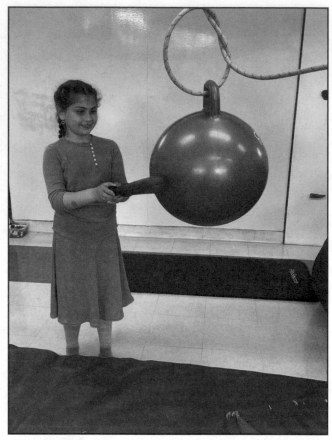

Figure 10-13.

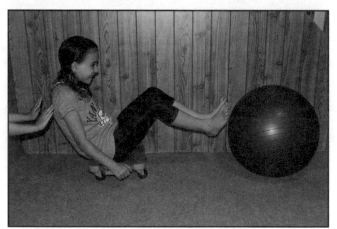

Figure 10-14.

- Child throws a small ball high up in the air and catches it. Upgrade this activity by performing it on a balance board.
- Child throws a ball against the wall and catches it without letting the ball drop on floor.
- Swing basketball: Therapist places a small basketball hoop next to a platform swing and places small bean bags or Koosh balls around the perimeter of the swing.

Child stands on the swing and picks up one piece at a time to throw into the basketball hoop. Therapist slowly swings the child back and forth; the child faces the direction of the basketball hoop while playing this game.

- Child sits upright on platform swing or on rolling scooter. Therapist pushes child toward a moving or stationary ball and child must kick ball upon initial contact (Figure 10-14).
- Child lies flat on back on floor. Therapist rolls large therapy ball toward child's feet. Child must kick ball when it comes near (Figures 10-15 and 10-16).
- Child lies on stomach on floor. Therapist rolls large therapy ball toward child. Child must push ball with hands when it comes near (Figures 10-17 through 10-19).
- Therapist or two children sit facing each other on floor with both legs completely extended and touching each other. Both children simultaneously turn feet in (position I; Figure 10-20) and then simultaneously turn feet out while slowly separating legs (position II; Figure 10-21). Therapist instructs child to maintain visual attention with feet throughout the activity.

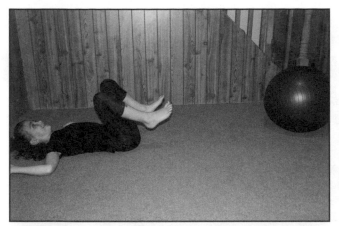

Figure 10-15.

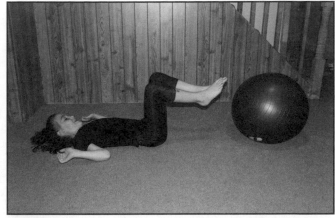

Figure 10-16.

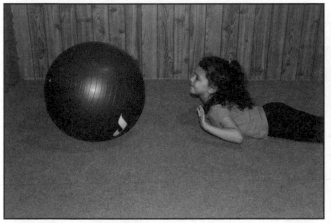

Figure 10-17.

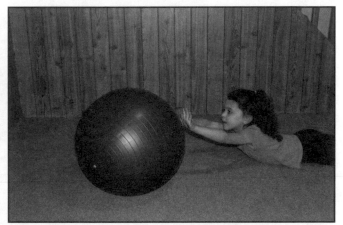

Figure 10-18.

- Two children lie prone, facing each other. They pass a ball to each other (Figures 10-22 and 10-23).

- Child goes into a tall kneel position. Therapist rolls large therapy ball toward child. Child must push ball away as it comes near.

- Children face each other, each holding balls. Children simultaneously throw ball at each other. Then repeat (Figures 10-24 and 10-25).

Online

- Visit www.eyecanlearn.com for additional visual scanning exercises.

- Visit www.abcteach.com and follow links for mazes and dot-to-dot handouts.

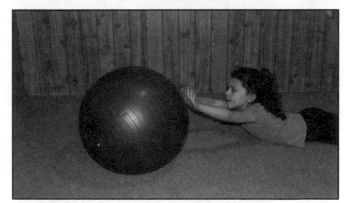

Figure 10-19.

Commercially Available Products

- Lucky Ducks
- Simon
- Whac-A-Mole
- Zoom Ball

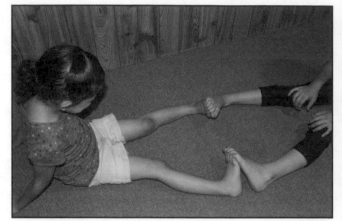

Figure 10-20.

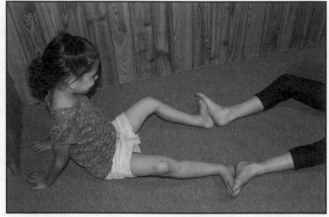

Figure 10-21.

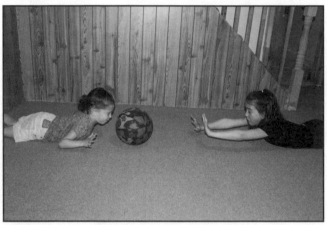

Figure 10-22.

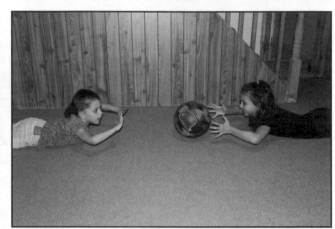

Figure 10-23.

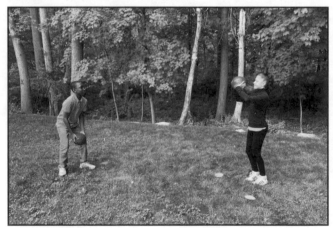

Figure 10-24.

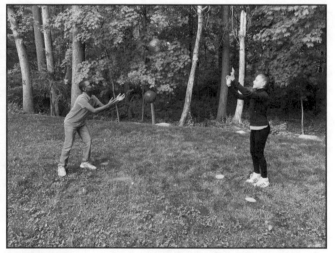

Figure 10-25.

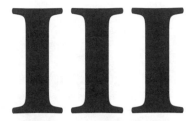

Dissociation Activities

The term *body dissociation* refers to the use of individual parts of the body in isolation from the rest of the body. When a child is unable to dissociate, their movements will appear stiff and clumsy. There are different forms of dissociation. In the upcoming chapters of this section, body dissociation and finger individuation are discussed.

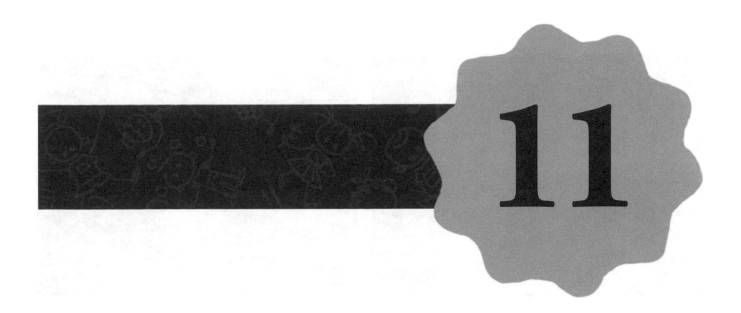

Body Dissociation

Body dissociation refers to the ability to move one part of the body without moving another part. For example, when rolling over, the child should be able to roll their body segmentally by dissociating the right and left extremities as well as the extremities and the head. A child with poor body dissociation will move stiffly—like a log—in one unit, as opposed to rolling segmentally (Tecklin, 2008).

Poor body dissociation may result in stiff, uncoordinated movement. This may also cause a child to use inefficient movement patterns, requiring more energy expenditure and taking more time. Additionally, postural control and reaching for objects is highly dependent on being able to segment and dissociate the different muscles of the trunk (Rachwani et al., 2015).

There are three main components to body dissociation: the ability to move parts of the upper body and lower body separately, the ability to move an extremity in isolation from the body and from the other extremity, and the ability to move the head and facial muscles in isolation from each other. This chapter provides activities to improve these three components of body dissociation.

This chapter also discusses exercises to work on torticollis. Torticollis is characterized by a tilting or turning of the head to one side (Hervey-Jumper et al., 2011). These exercises are provided in the present chapter because a child

with tight neck muscles will have difficulty dissociating their head and neck from the rest of the body and may subsequently present with difficulties in overall dissociation.

BODY DISSOCIATION TREATMENT ACTIVITIES

Whole Body Dissociation

- Baseball: Therapist places a baseball or Wiffle Ball on a tee. Child swings the bat to hit the ball off the tee. Although this game can also be played without a tee, it will be easier to work on dissociating the different trunk muscles if the ball is hit off the tee in a slow, controlled fashion (as opposed to swinging at a ball in the air).

- Place child (developmentally 6 to 14 months; Cottrell, 2004, p. 19) on side and place a toy in front of child to motivate them to roll over fully (Figure 11-1).

- Twist child's legs toward side to be rolled in order to give child a head start (Figure 11-2).

Danto, A. H., & Pruzansky, M. *1001 Pediatric Treatment Activities: Creative Ideas for Therapy Sessions, Third Edition* (pp. 73-77).

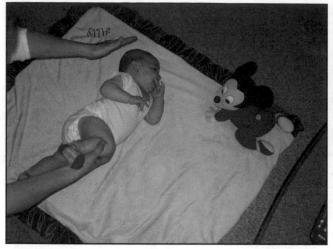

Figure 11-1.

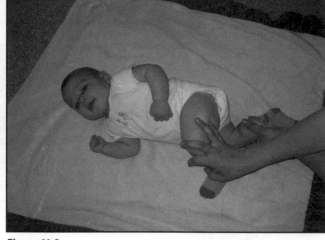

Figure 11-2.

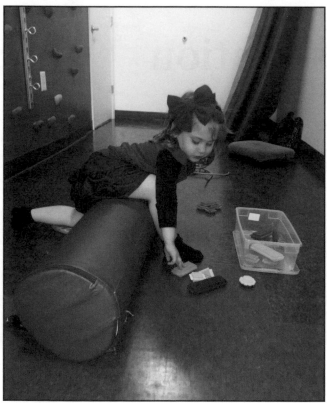

Figure 11-3.

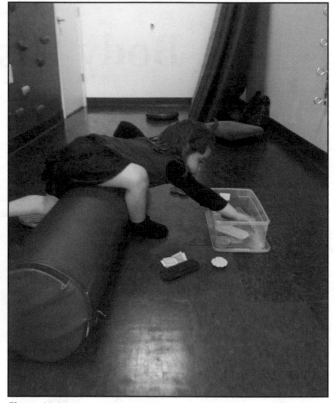

Figure 11-4.

- Rolling: Child slowly rolls on a mat segmentally (first head, then trunk, then legs)—not like a log. If child appears stiff while rolling, therapist can provide child with verbal and physical cuing as needed.

- Fast running: Child runs across the room or outside. Therapist can remind child to utilize an arm swing when running.

- Frog jump activities: Child squats down on the floor and frog jumps as far as possible. Child jumps to a basket and places Koosh balls or other toys in it to make this activity more playful.

- Child faces large bolster and places one leg over bolster and other leg in kneeling position. Child reaches for objects on both sides and places them in the container (Figures 11-3 and 11-4).

- Mother holds child with one knee bent/hip flexed in front of mother's stomach, other leg straight and relaxed behind mother's back.

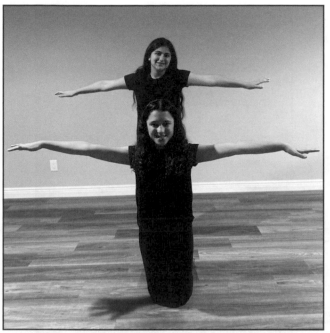

Figure 11-5.

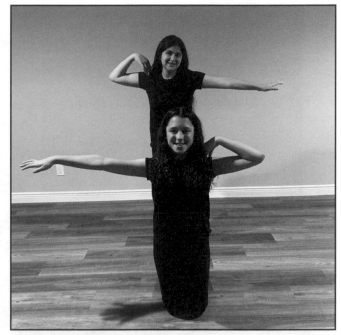

Figure 11-6.

Dissociating Extremities From the Body

- Dry-wet game: Therapist wets different parts of child's body with water, alternating between wetting a part on the child's right side and left side (e.g., arms, fingers, shoulders, knees). Therapist calls out a body part that is wet ("wet hand") and child must extend/raise only the body part that is wet while keeping the dry body part down.

- Child moves both arms three to four times in a specific direction (in and out, up and down, to the side, etc.). Therapist then asks child to move only one side in that same direction and motion. This game can also be played with the lower extremities.

  ○ Position 1 (Figure 11-5), Position 2 (Figure 11-6), Position 3 (Figure 11-7).

- Child lies on floor or stands against the wall. Child lifts one leg or arm at a time off the floor or wall while keeping the other limb flush against the resting surface.

- Child stands still with both hands on hips and kicks a moving ball.

- Child shrugs one shoulder at a time.

- Child lies on floor or outdoors in snow and makes snow angels. Child then attempts to do this using only on one side at a time.

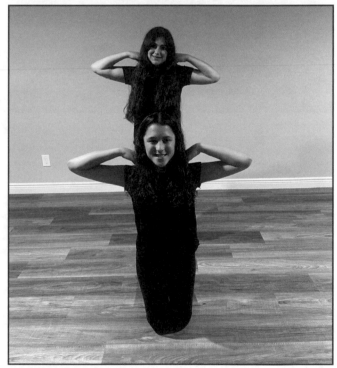

Figure 11-7.

- Child turns a jump rope with one hand (therapist can tie a rope to a doorknob or hold the other end of the rope) while keeping the rest of the body still (Figure 11-8).

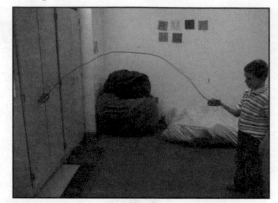

Figure 11-8.

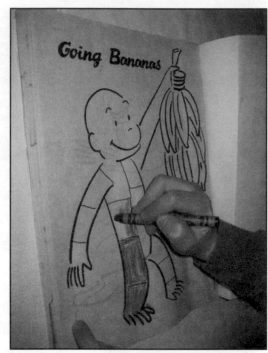

Figure 11-9.

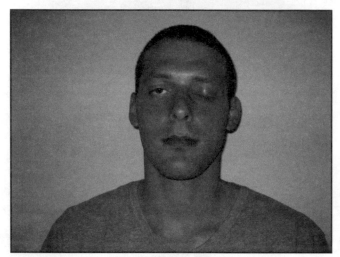

Figure 11-10.

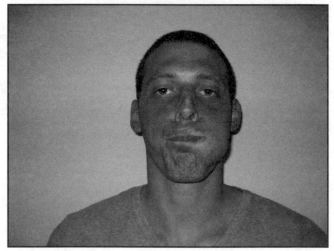

Figure 11-11.

- Coloring activity: To help a child use isolated wrist/ finger movements instead of whole arm movements in coloring a large picture, therapist can divide a picture into many smaller sections. If the child is able to follow instructions and color in only one section at a time, this will automatically cause the child to use more isolated movements (Figure 11-9).

Dissociating Head and Facial Muscles

- Child visually tracks a moving target while keeping the head still.

- Child shakes head "yes" and "no" without moving the shoulders or any part of the trunk.

- Child moves head all around in a circle, keeping the rest of the body still.

- Child moves one side of the facial muscles at a time to wink, close an eye, blow up one cheek, or move the lips. Child then switches and makes the same movements using only the muscles on the other side of the face (Figures 11-10 and 11-11).

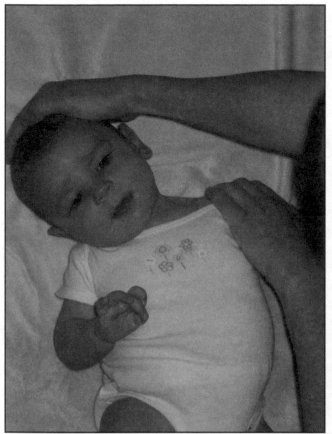

Figure 11-12.

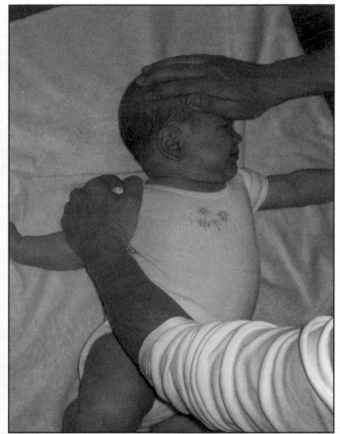

Figure 11-13.

Treating Torticollis

- Massage child's tight neck muscles with lotion.
- Elongate and stretch child's tight neck muscles (Figures 11-12 and 11-13).

Do not perform any stretches on child without first being taught how to properly handle and stretch child by either a doctor or a trained occupational or physical therapist. Repeat at each diaper change.

- Have child face the nonpreferred side: Stimulate this by either placing a toy on the nonpreferred side for child to look at or having an adult play Peek-a-Boo on nonpreferred side. Child can be sitting, lying on back, belly, or on your lap (Figure 11-14).

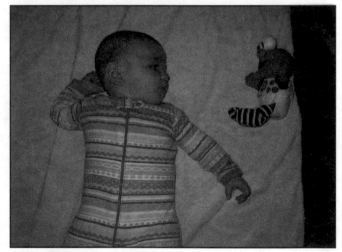

Figure 11-14.

- Place stroller toys toward the nonpreferred side of the child during walks.
- When child is sleeping, turn child's head to nonpreferred side.
- Have child play in side-lying position.

- Increase tummy time. See Chapter 20, "Upper Arm Strengthening and Stabilization," for ways to help increase child's tolerance of tummy time.
- Therapist or parent holds baby on adult's hip on the side that forces the baby to turn head in direction that causes a stretch to tight neck muscles.

Finger Individuation

Finger individuation is the ability to move a single finger in isolation from the other fingers. Being able to individuate the digits is one of the hallmarks of human motor control (Thielbar et al., 2014). Relatively independent finger movements rely on the motor cortex and the corticospinal tract (Lemon et al., 1986). The anatomy and structure of the hand's internal bones, muscles, tendons, and ligaments allow for an unlimited combination of varied movements (Benbow, 1997). Movements of the fingers occur over multiple joints causing coactivation of noninvolved joints (Jones & Lederman, 2006). The accurate coordination of finger movements is also necessary in order to approximate the size, shape, and use of an object before making contact with it (Raghavan et al., 2007). Some children are unable to move an individual finger in isolation from the other fingers and, therefore, cannot master the level of precision needed for fine motor activities.

This chapter provides activities that require isolated finger use and can help promote improved hand and finger function.

FINGER INDIVIDUATION TREATMENT ACTIVITIES

Playful Finger Games

- Child sings "Where Is Thumpkin?" while holding up the appropriate finger:

    Where is Thumpkin, where is Thumpkin?
    Chorus:
    Here I am, here I am.
    How are you today sir?
    Very well I thank you.
    Run away, run away.

    ○ Follow with "pointer," "tall man," "ring man," and "pinky."

- Therapist and child play "This Little Piggy": In playing this game, child sticks out one finger at a time (Figure 12-1).

- Counting: Child counts out loud with fingers, one number at a time. Child counts forward to 10 and then backward.

Danto, A. H., & Pruzansky, M. *1001 Pediatric Treatment Activities: Creative Ideas for Therapy Sessions, Third Edition* (pp. 79-82).
© 2023 SLACK Incorporated.

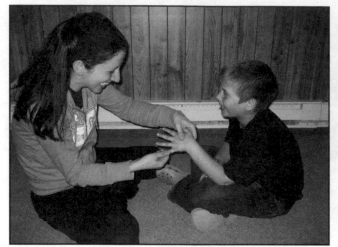

Figure 12-1.

- Therapist places finger puppets on child's fingers. Child then acts out a story.

- Thumb wars.

This game should be played only between therapist and child, not between two children, to make sure that no one gets hurt.

- Therapist teaches child basic sign language signs and how to sign the alphabet in sign language.

Computer and Keyboard Activities

- Child plays computer games that involve pushing specific buttons with specific fingers.

- Child plays computer games that require use of a mouse: Many children have difficulty using a mouse because they are unable to push down with their index fingers in isolation and instead push down with both fingers together.

- Typing: Using the keyboard keys, child writes words and sentences or a story.

- Child plays a song on a piano or keyboard. If this is too challenging, child can copy/imitate hitting specific notes on the piano.

Crafts and Coloring

- Finger crayons
  - Therapist places a different finger crayon on each of child's fingers. Child colors a picture with finger crayons.

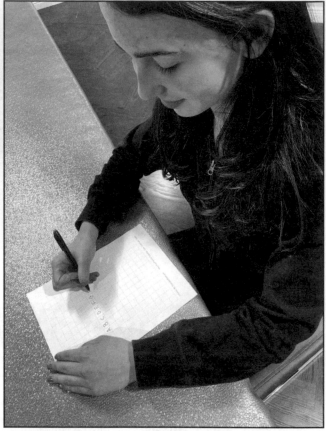

Figure 12-2.

  - Therapist places finger crayons on each of child's fingers. Therapist tells child to make a line, but only with a specific color. Therapist then asks child to make a line by using two colors together at the same time.

- Child peels stickers off of a sticker sheet and places the stickers on a piece of paper.

- Child colors in or traces gradually smaller shapes.

- Bead games: Therapist places a small bead between the child's index finger and thumb. Child rolls the bead back and forth and from side to side. Child then transfers bead between the next finger and thumb and performs the same activity. Child continues to the pinky and then works back toward the thumb.

- Play-Doh/Theraputty: Child pushes one finger at a time down into the putty.

- Child strings beads to make a necklace.

- Child crumples small pieces of tissue paper with one hand, using only the fingertips to crumple the paper.

- Child writes letters in small graph paper boxes (Figures 12-2 and 12-3).

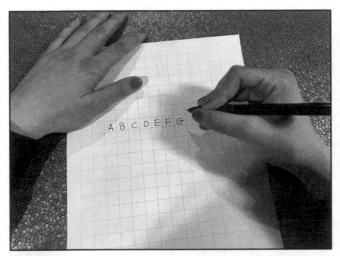

Figure 12-3.

Finger Exercises and Positions

- Child touches each finger to the thumb one at a time (Figure 12-4).

- Child imitates different hand and finger positions.

- Finger writing: Child pretends that their fingertip is a pencil and writes a word on a piece of paper using only the fingertip. Therapist may need to gently stabilize child's hand so that only the finger and the fingertips move to write the letters. (This activity may be difficult for some children and some may resist using fine finger movements. The supervising therapist should use only gentle guidance in assisting any child in this activity.)

- Child carries multiple items in each hand. Child uses the fingers to wrap around each item (around a loop, bag strap, Hula Hoop, pen, or anything that can be gripped with just the fingers). Therapist calls out one item, and child must release that item without dropping other items in their hand. An alternative way to play this game is with paper. Child holds colored strips of construction paper between each finger. Therapist calls out a color, and child must drop the specific color without releasing any other color (Figures 12-5 and 12-6).

- Child pushes a finger popping toy using one finger at a time and alternates fingers (Figure 12-7).

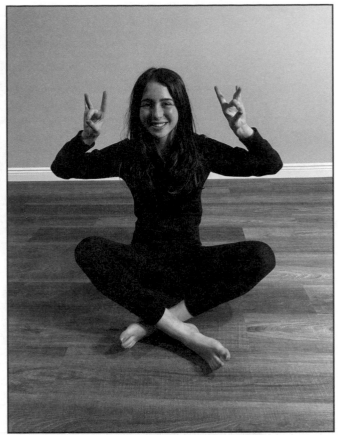

Figure 12-4.

Using the Thumb and Index Finger Together

- Child picks up small pellet-sized objects.

- Page turning: Child turns the pages of a storybook, one page at a time.

- Card dealing: Child deals out a deck of cards using only one hand at a time, thereby forcing the child to isolate thumb movements in dealing out the cards.

- Child twirls a pen around the fingers.

- Spin a top: Child practices spinning a top on a tabletop, floor, or other hard surface.

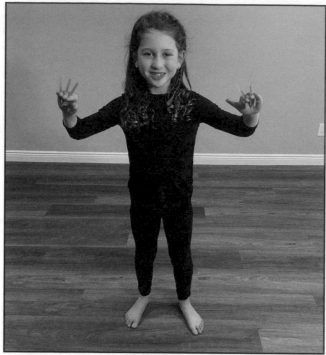

Figure 12-5.

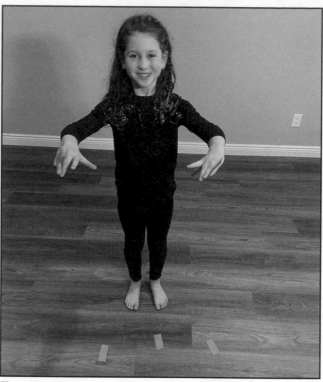

Figure 12-6.

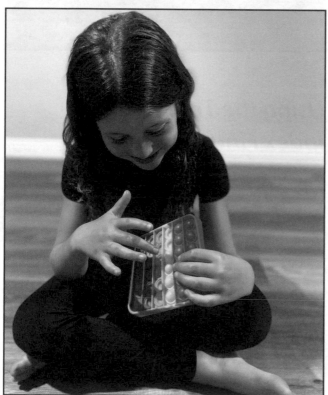

Figure 12-7.

Playing Musical Instruments

- Therapist teaches child some notes or chords on any instrument with strings, including guitar, violin, and cello (Figure 12-8).

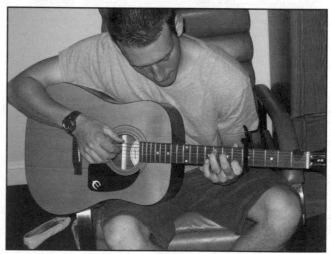

Figure 12-8.

- Therapist teaches child some notes or chords on any instrument with buttons or holes to press or cover, including recorder, horn instruments, and brass instruments.

Commercially Available Product

- Etch A Sketch

IV

Hand Skills

Hand skills are needed for everyday functioning with gross motor tasks as well as tasks involving fine precision. This section includes activities that can assist in improving functional hand use by focusing on the necessary prerequisites needed. It also focuses on placing the hand and fingers in the correct position when engaged in a fine motor activity and playing games with very small objects that require precision. Finally, it focuses on strengthening the small muscles of the hand as well as practicing skills that involve those muscles, such as grasping a sock to pull it on, coloring with a crayon, or engaging in craft activities. It is important to understand typical development of various hand and other fine motor skills in order to select appropriate treatment activities and when establishing goals (Exner, 1997).

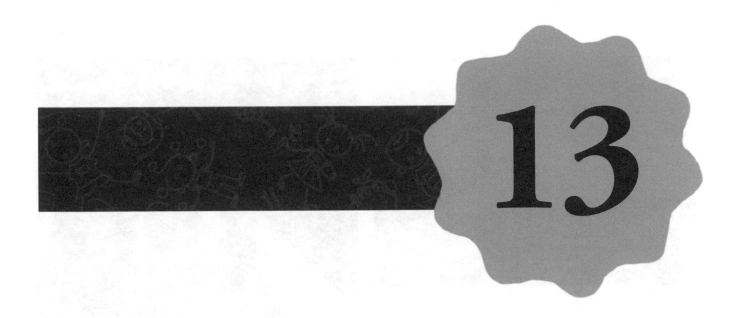

Open Webspace

An open webspace (Figure 13-1) is the space between the thumb and the index finger that appears when grasping an object; the index finger is in proper opposition with the thumb. When the webspace is closed (i.e., when using a lateral pencil grasp) there is an associated increase in whole arm movement and upper back muscle activation (Farris et al., 2019). Consequently, there is a resulting decrease in dynamic finger movements. Pencil grasps using a lateral grasp where a closed webspace is typically present, will negatively affect handwriting, especially in boys (Farris et al., 2019).

This chapter provides two types of activities. First, there are activities that promote moving the fingers to the tip of the thumb, promoting opposition and thereby opening the webspace. The second type of activity involves wrapping the child's hands around different objects, naturally creating an open webspace. The activities provided in this chapter are intended to help a child promote the finger and hand stability needed for precision and fine motor skills.

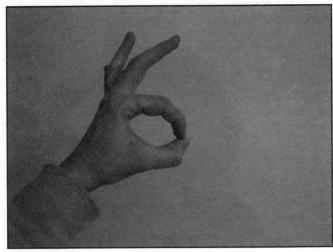

Figure 13-1.

Danto, A. H., & Pruzansky, M. *1001 Pediatric Treatment Activities: Creative Ideas for Therapy Sessions, Third Edition* (pp. 85-88).

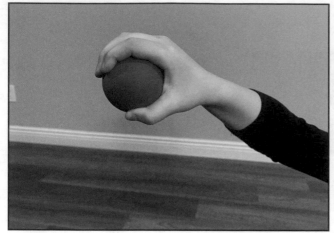

Figure 13-2.

ACTIVITIES TO OPEN THE WEBSPACE

Exercises

- Child touches each finger to the thumb, going forward, backward, and then on both hands simultaneously.

- Making "Os": Child practices forming the letter "O" with the webspace.

- Stretching exercises: Therapist gently massages and then stretches the webspace open for the child.

- Finger Twister: Therapist creates a mini Twister board and has child play Twister with the fingers.

- Child places hand on table and then makes wide circles with thumb. Repeat circles 20 times. Therapist may need to stabilize digits two to five if child is unable to keep hand still.

- Finger Painting "Os": Therapist places finger paint on child's thumb. Child draws "Os" with thumb while keeping other fingers flat on the paper.

- Child picks up small pellet-sized beads while keeping hand in shape of an "O" and then releases them into container.

- Child holds mini marshmallow between index finger and thumb while fingers are positioned around marshmallow in shape of an "O." Child holds marshmallow gently so as to not crush it and slowly counts to 10 while maintaining position.

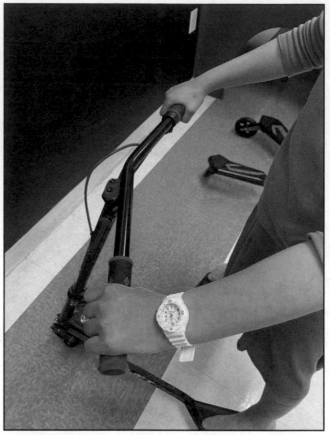

Figure 13-3.

- Child slides pencil or marker up and down tips of fingers with only one hand (i.e., child "walks" fingers up and down the pencil).

Special Equipment

- Child uses different pencil grippers in writing or coloring to help keep the webspace open during activities with a writing utensil.

Wrapping the Hands Around Round Objects

- Wrap hand around the following:
  - Small balls (Figure 13-2).
  - Handles on a bike (Figure 13-3).
  - Rungs on a ladder in the playground.

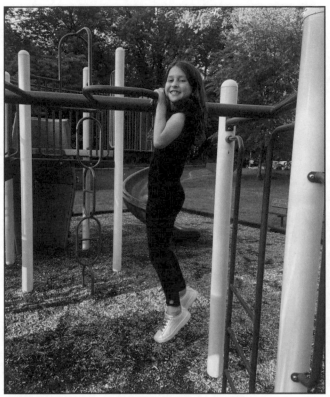

Figure 13-4.

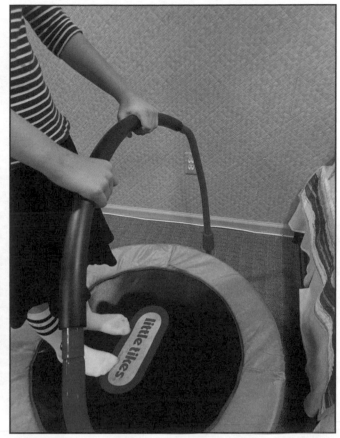

Figure 13-5.

- ○ Rungs on the monkey bars in a playground (Figure 13-4).
- ○ Around trampoline handlebars (Figure 13-5).
- ○ Around jump rope handles (Figure 13-6).
- Use a roller to flatten dough.
- Hold onto ropes while on platform swing.
- Hold onto trapeze bar (Figure 13-7).
- Sit on seesaw and hold onto handlebars.
- Child holds pencil with proper grasp while therapist encourages an open webspace (Figure 13-8).

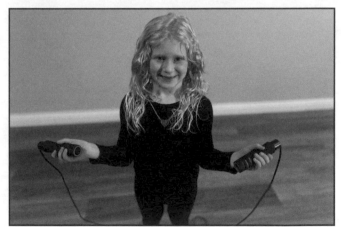

Figure 13-6.

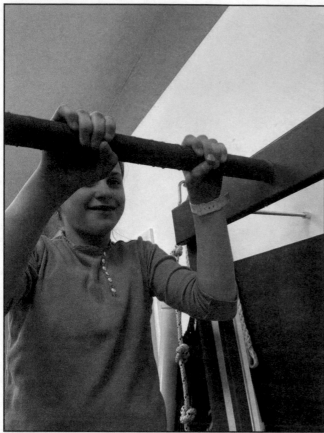

Figure 13-7.

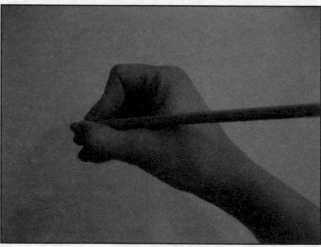

Figure 13-8.

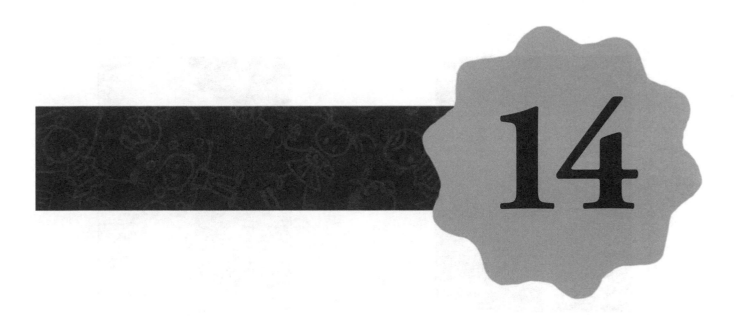

Fine Motor Skills

Acquiring fine motor skills is a critical component of child development. These skills allow children to participate in valued occupations including activities of daily living, learning, and playing (Marr et al., 2003). There is also a strong relationship between in-hand manipulation skills and handwriting proficiency (Cornhill & Case-Smith, 1996). Children who struggle with fine motor skills risk falling behind in school, becoming dependent on others, and getting teased in school. (Losse et al., 1991; Piek et al., 2006). There is also research to indicate that occupational therapy intervention dealing with fine motor skills is effective in preschool and lower elementary school. (Bazyk et al., 2009).

The present chapter provides activities that will help to strengthen fine motor skills by engaging a child in games and activities with small parts and pieces. The purpose of the suggested activities is to improve overall manual dexterity. The activities provided require a child to use in-hand manipulation, pincer grasp, and other manipulative skills.

FINE MOTOR ACTIVITIES

Theraputty/Play-Doh

- Child makes little balls out of Theraputty or Play-Doh by rolling small pieces between the fingertips. Child then picks up pieces with tongs and places them into a nearby container.

- Child finds the letters of their name on letter beads. Child then hides those specific letter beads in Theraputty or Play-Doh and subsequently finds them.

Writing/Coloring

- Finger crayons: Child colors and makes a picture with finger crayons placed on specific fingers (Figures 14-1 and 14-2).

- Toothpicks activity: Therapist traces child's name lightly on a piece of Styrofoam board with a pencil or pen. Child places toothpicks, one at a time, into Styrofoam along the traced letters of name to poke holes (Figure 14-3). Child then colors over the letters (Figure 14-4).

Danto, A. H., & Pruzansky, M. *1001 Pediatric Treatment Activities: Creative Ideas for Therapy Sessions, Third Edition* (pp. 89-94).

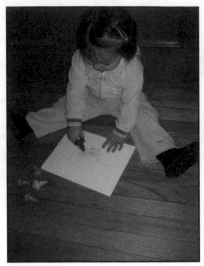

Figure 14-1.

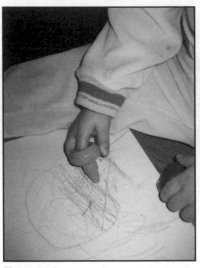

Figure 14-2.

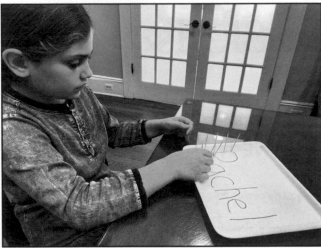

Figure 14-3.

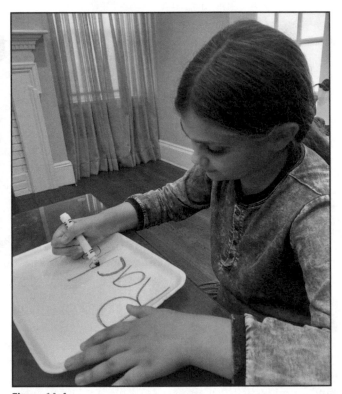

Figure 14-4.

Beading and Lacing Activities

- Pop Beads
  - Child pushes and connects small Pop Beads together, then pulls them apart one at a time (Figures 14-5 and 14-6).
  - Child pushes and connects large Pop Beads together, then pulls them apart one at a time (Figures 14-7 and 14-8).
- Food art: Child strings macaroni to make a necklace, bracelet, or another design.
- Froot Loops necklace: Child strings Froot Loops on a long, thin piece of licorice (this activity can also be performed with Cheerios).

- Lacing beads: Child strings beads on a thin piece of string. (If this is too challenging, this activity can be downgraded by stringing the beads onto a pipe cleaner.)
- Bead rolling: Therapist places a small bead between child's index finger and thumb. Child rolls the bead back and forth, from side to side, and then in circles. Child then tries to transfer bead between the next finger and thumb and perform the same activity. Child continues to the pinky and works back toward the thumb.

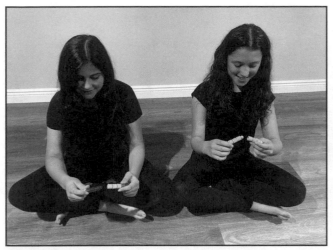

Figure 14-5.

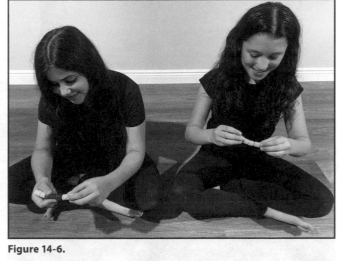

Figure 14-6.

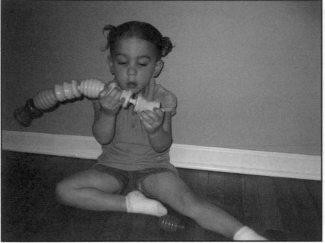

Figure 14-7.

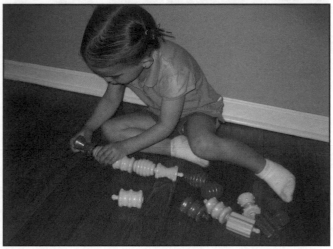

Figure 14-8.

- Lacing art and sewing kits: Therapist teaches child different sewing stitches (whip stitch/over-under stitch) with a needle and thread. (Make sure the needle is not too sharp and that this activity is performed only with a child having appropriate safety awareness.)

Peeling With the Fingertips

- Child peels strips of masking tape off a tape roll. Child makes shapes, letters, or a picture with the strips. (This activity is often more fun for a child when colored masking tape is used.)
- Child peels stickers off of a sticker sheet and places them on a piece of paper.
- Button Candy: Therapist gives child a reward of Button Candy and asks child to peel the candy off the sheet of paper (Figure 14-9).
- Turning pages: Therapist reads child a book. Child turns the pages with fingertips.

- Pop-up books: Therapist reads child a pop-up book. Child lifts tabs off the page with their fingertips.
- Child peels an orange or grapefruit and is then allowed to eat it.
- Cookie cutters: Child pushes cookie cutter into dough and then peels out cookie shape by pulling away excess dough.

Manipulating Small Objects

- Grasp-release activities (developmental age 7 to 9 months)
  - Therapist places toy fish in a small toy fishbowl and has child take all of the fish out of fishbowl and then put them back in one at a time. (The Ocean Wonders Musical Fishbowl plays music to reinforce putting in and taking out the fish, which may make this activity more reinforcing to the child.)

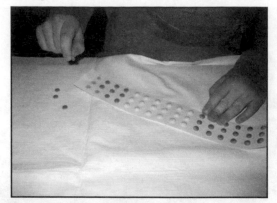

Figure 14-9.

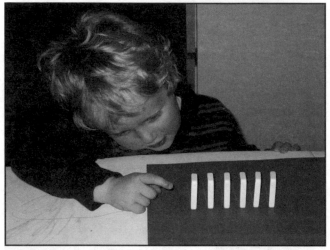

Figure 14-11.

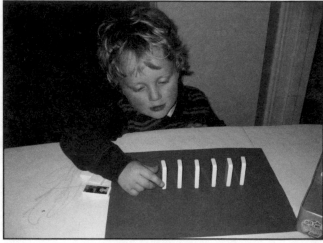

Figure 14-10.

- Penny picture handouts: Child picks up one penny at a time and places the pennies onto the circular marks on the penny flipping handout to make a design. (See Appendix A, pp. 242-244, for sample penny handouts.)
- Child breaks pistachio shells off and gets to eat the nut inside.

Be sure to check for nut allergy.

Cutting Activities

- Therapist draws lines, shapes, or pictures of animals on a piece of paper. Child practices cutting along the lines to cut out the picture. If this is too challenging, therapist can hold a 1-inch strip of paper and allow child to make snips in the paper. (See Appendix A, pp. 197-202, for sample cutting activity pages.)

Keys

- Lock and key: Therapist provides child with different keys. Child unlocks different doors or locked boxes.
- Child adds keys onto a key chain ring. (The larger the key chain ring, the easier the activity.)

Games

- Therapist demonstrates "cause and effect" toy where the child has to press/pull/push a knob or button to make a character pop up (developmental age of 6 to 9 months).
- Dominoes: Child creates a long line of dominoes on a flat surface and then tips the last domino to watch the "domino effect." It may be necessary to help child with this task to make sure that no dominoes are accidentally knocked over too early (Figures 14-10 through 14-12).

- ○ Therapist takes a simple bucket and several toys that the child enjoys playing with. Therapist places toys in the bucket. The child removes the toys one at a time and then places them back in the bucket. Repeat several times.
- Child attaches paper clips in a chain.
- Nuts and bolts: Child screws together nuts and bolts of different sizes.
- Therapist scatters several pennies/coins on table. Child picks up three coins, one at a time. Child places each coin, one at a time, back into a piggy bank (to upgrade this activity to work on in-hand manipulation and translation, increase the number of pennies the child must pick up at one time).
- Penny flipping: Therapist places 10 pennies on the table in a line. Child turns each penny over, one at a time.
- Penny design making: Child creates different pictures and designs using pennies.

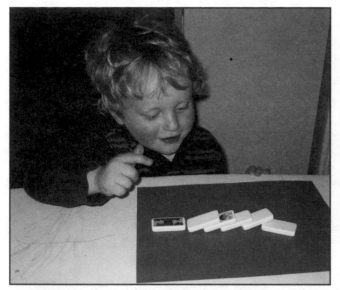

Figure 14-12.

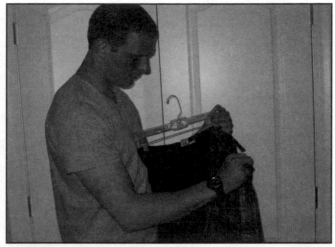

Figure 14-13.

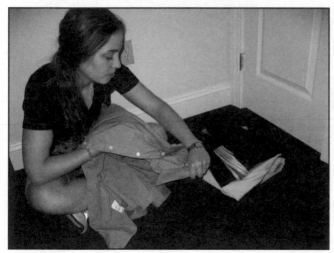

Figure 14-14.

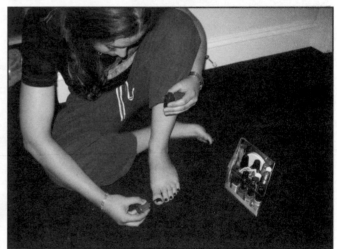

Figure 14-15.

- Card flipping: Therapist plays a card game or a game of Memory in which child must flip cards over on the table. (Do not let the child drag the card to the edge of the table to flip it or else they will not be using the small muscles in the fingers for the card-flipping task.)

- Travel-sized games: Child plays travel-sized games with small pieces (some examples include Checkers, Chess, and Connect Four).

Dressing and Grooming

- Doll dressing: Child plays with small dolls, dressing and undressing them.

- Dressing skills and manipulating fasteners. Child can engage in the following:

  ○ Tying and untying shoelaces

  ○ Buttoning and unbuttoning a shirt

  ○ Buckling and unbuckling belt buckles

  ○ Zipping and unzipping zippers

  ○ Snapping and unsnapping snaps

  ○ Hooking overall latches and unhooking

- Don't drop the clothes: Therapist places many skirts or pants on a skirt hanger. Child tries to hold hanger up in the air and remove one article of clothing from the hanger without letting the others fall to the floor (Figure 14-13).

- Folding activities: Therapist teaches child how to fold clothing neatly in a pile (Figure 14-14).

- Makeup application: Therapist teaches older children how to apply makeup.

- Nail polish: Therapist and child practice polishing fingernails or toenails (Figure 14-15).

Commercially Available Products

- ADL books
- Bead art
- *The Cheerios Play Book*
- Connect Four
- Cootie

- Don't Spill the Beans
- Hi Ho Cherry-O
- Lite Brite
- Mancala
- Mastermind
- Melissa & Doug Basic Skills Board
- Melissa & Doug Latches Puzzle
- Perler Beads
- Tinkertoys

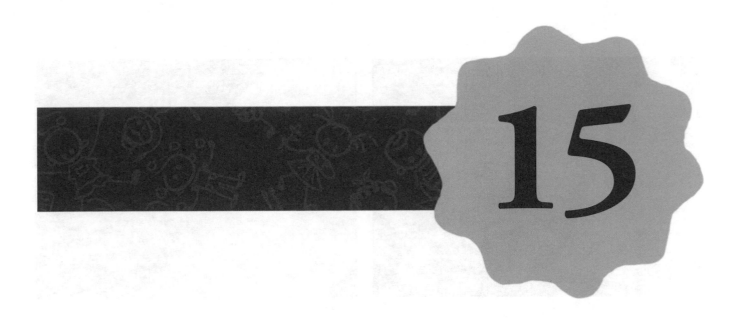

Pinch-Grasp Manipulation

A pincer grasp involves gripping an item between the thumb and index finger and typically emerges at 9 months of age (Gerber et al., 2010). Adequate pinch-grasp strength is required for many activities of daily living, including eating and playing. Many children with various disabilities will demonstrate decreased pincer grasp strength (Häger-Ross & Rösblad, 2002). The present chapter discusses ways to work on strengthening the pinch-grasp.

PINCH-GRASP MANIPULATION

Pincer Activities

- Child colors with small broken pieces of crayons (Figure 15-1). This automatically places child's fingers in correct pincer position for coloring and prewriting activities.
- Child colors with adapted pencil grips and graspers placed on writing utensil (Figure 15-2).
- Child picks up small, pellet-sized items (e.g., beads, small cubes, rice).
- Child picks up pennies to place into piggy bank.

- Child uses tongs, chopsticks, or tweezers to pick up small objects. Suggested objects to pick up include marshmallows, Styrofoam, nuts, beads, and pom-poms (note: the closer to the tip the child holds the tong, the easier the activity becomes).
- Child places toothpicks deep into resistive Theraputty to make a picture of a smiley face, a flower, a circle, etc. Child then removes each toothpick one at a time.
- Tissue paper projects: Child cuts up small strips of tissue paper. Child crumples each piece of tissue paper and then glues it to a paper to make a picture or create a letter of their name (Figure 15-3).
- Tissue paper butterfly: Child crumbles small pieces of cut-up tissue paper in each hand, holding hands in the air when crumbling and not against body. Child places pieces on a butterfly to decorate (Figure 15-4).
- Stringing beads: Child laces beads to make a necklace. To downgrade this activity, the child can string beads onto a pipe cleaner instead of a string.
- Bead rolling: Therapist scatters beads on the table. Child picks up a bead one at a time and squeezes it between the index finger and thumb and holds for 3 seconds. Child then rolls bead back and forth, side to side, and then transfers it into a cup.

Danto, A. H., & Pruzansky, M. *1001 Pediatric Treatment Activities:*
Creative Ideas for Therapy Sessions, Third Edition (pp. 95-98).
© 2023 SLACK Incorporated.

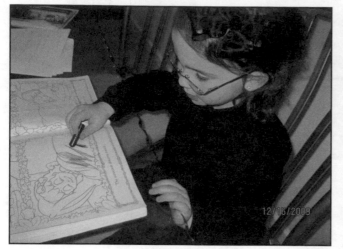

Figure 15-1.

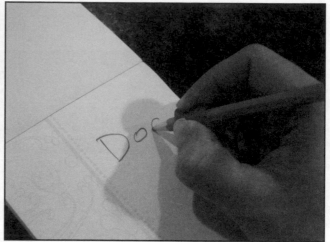

Figure 15-2.

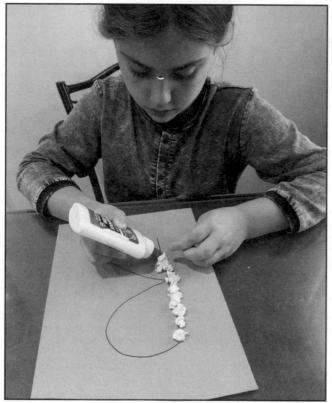

Figure 15-3.

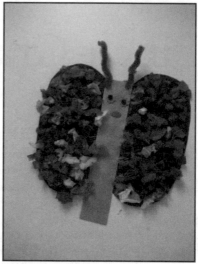

Figure 15-4.

- Stamps: Child picks up different stamps with small handles and stamps a paper or their own skin.

- Stickers: Therapist draws a picture of a smiley face or something else the child likes. Child puts very small stickers on the lines of the drawing and on the eyes, nose, mouth, etc.

- Child squeezes toothpick between thumb and index finger and sticks toothpick into various small marshmallows or pieces of fruit and eats them.

Pincer Strengthening

- Child uses a reacher to pick up items off the floor and places them into a bucket (Figure 15-8).

- Child completes clothespin activities.

  o Child places clothespins on string to make a necklace.

- Play-Doh rolling: Child rolls pellet-sized balls of Play-Doh between the thumb and pointer finger, then squeezes them one by one using a pinch-grasp.

- Small knobbed puzzles: Child holds the small knob on the puzzle piece to complete the puzzle (Figure 15-5).

- Magna Doodle boards: Child holds the small tips of the Magna Doodle pieces to color a picture (Figures 15-6 and 15-7).

- Wind-up toys: Child winds up different wind-up toys and watches them go.

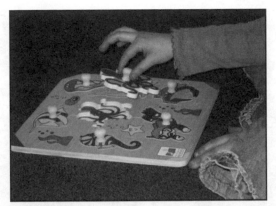

Figure 15-5.

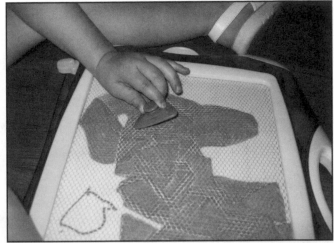

Figure 15-6.

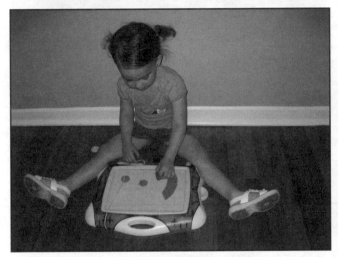

Figure 15-7.

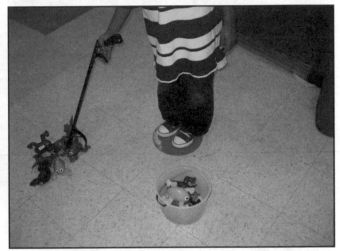

Figure 15-8.

- ○ Therapist writes letters on clothespins and has child form words with clothespins (Figures 15-9 and 15-10).
- Spray water bottles: Child helps water plants or washes off the chalkboard with a spray water bottle.
- Water guns: Therapist fills a water gun with water and creates a bull's-eye to be placed on the wall. Child stands a few feet away from the target and squirts the water at the bull's-eye.
- Gluing activities: Child squeezes a glue bottle with the thumb and index fingers.

- Bubble Wrap: Child pinches individual bubbles on Bubble Wrap between thumb and index finger.
- Sponge activities
  - ○ Child squeezes small sponges for sponge painting.
  - ○ Child wets small sponges and erases letters on a chalkboard (Figure 15-11).

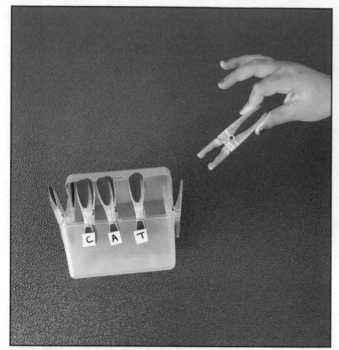

Figure 15-9.

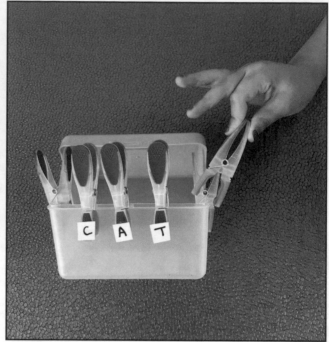

Figure 15-10.

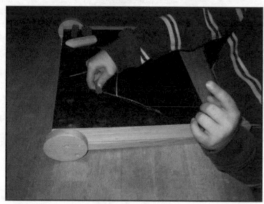

Figure 15-11.

Commercially Available Products

- Ants in the Pants
- Barbecue Party
- Bed Bugs
- Design and Drill Activity Center

- Digi-Piggy Digital Piggy Bank
- Digital Coin Bank
- Gator Grabber Tweezers
- Hungry Dog/Monkey/Bunny Motor Skills Game
- Hungry Hungry Hippos
- Jolly Octopus
- Mr. Mouth
- Operation
- Peg Domino
- Plastic Jumping Frog Toys
- Rock Em' Sock Em' Robots
- Scatterpillar Scramble
- Squiggly Worms
- Super Sorting Pie
- Tiddlywinks
- Wok 'N Roll

Hand Strengthening

Adequate fine motor skills (as mentioned in previous chapters) are only part of what is needed for functional hand use. Sufficient grip strength is necessary for independence with various activities of daily living (Häger-Ross & Rösblad, 2002). Grip strength may significantly influence a child's performance in various activities of daily living. Increased grip strength has also been shown to correlate with improved pencil control and improved handwriting in typically developing children (Alaniz et al., 2015). Increasing the strength of the hand can also help a child better control fine motor movements (Huffman & Fortenberry, 2011).

Measurements of grip strength are often used in treatment planning (Häger-Ross & Rösblad, 2002). This chapter not only provides activities to increase hand strength but also focuses on endurance as an equally important principle.

HAND-STRENGTHENING ACTIVITIES

Push and Pull

- LEGO pieces: Child pushes LEGO pieces together tightly and then pulls them apart.
- Pop Beads
  - Therapist holds chain of Pop Beads and allows child to pull beads off the other end.
  - Child pushes together Pop Beads and then pulls apart one bead at a time.
- Rapper Snappers: Therapist crunches up a Rapper Snapper toy and holds one end while child grasps the other end. Therapist encourages the child to pull one way while the therapist pulls the other way (the noise that this toy makes when being stretched is very reinforcing).

Danto, A. H., & Pruzansky, M. *1001 Pediatric Treatment Activities: Creative Ideas for Therapy Sessions, Third Edition* (pp. 99-102).

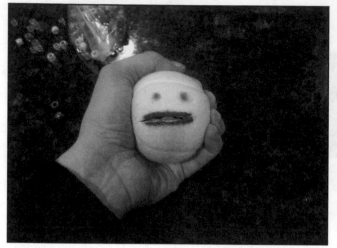

Figure 16-1.

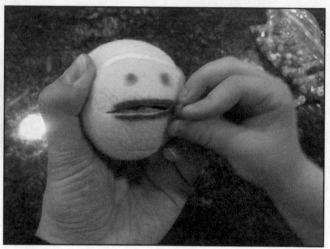

Figure 16-2.

Squeezing and Pinching

- Tennis ball smiley face: To create this, the therapist or child draws a smiley face on a tennis ball and then an adult uses scissors or a knife to cut a 1-inch slit in the tennis ball over the mouth. Child then squeezes the sides of the tennis ball to place in small beads. After child completes placing the beads in ball, the child can make the tennis ball have a stomach ache and "throw up" all the beads (Figures 16-1 and 16-2). (The larger the slit on the tennis ball, the easier the activity.)

- Theraputty exercises

  ○ Child pinches, pulls, and squeezes Theraputty.

  ○ Child hides different objects in putty and then finds them as quickly as possible. (This activity can be made more exciting by using a timer to see how quickly child can work and then see if child can break their record.)

- Play-Doh

  ○ Child rolls and squeezes Play-Doh.

  ○ Child creates different objects, including a ball, square, and triangle, with the Play-Doh.

- Knead dough: Child helps prepare dough for a baking activity and kneads dough until it is smooth.

- Squeeze toys: Child squeezes a stress ball, Koosh ball, or another sensory ball.

- Using resistive grippers: Child performs hand-strengthening exercises on a hand gripper (Figures 16-3 and 16-4). Add rubber bands to increase resistance as needed.

- Puff paint: Child squeezes puff paint onto a paper, a fabric, or another craft surface of choice to draw a picture or make a design.

- Squeezing glue: Child squeezes glue out of a container onto a line. (Be sure to use glue out of a container and not a glue stick.) This can be incorporated into any gluing and pasting craft activity of choice.

- Child fills a squeeze toy with water and shoots it.

- Pustefix Bubble Bear: Child maintains a continuous squeeze on the bottle to keep the wand up out of the bottle and blows bubbles (Figure 16-5).

Increasing Endurance

- Hand puppets: Child performs a play with different hand puppets.

- Coloring: Child colors in large pictures in coloring books.

- Snapping fingers: Therapist teaches child how to snap fingers together; they then snap along together to a song.

- Hand exercises: Child opens and closes hand and fingers to the beat of a song.

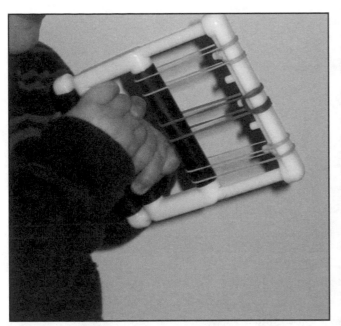

Figure 16-3.

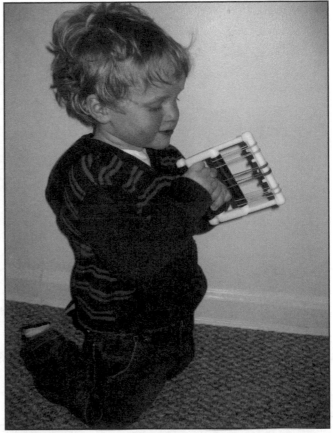

Figure 16-4.

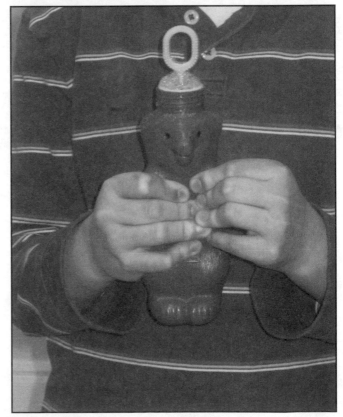

Figure 16-5.

Cutting Activities

- Simple cutting: Therapist draws lines, shapes, or animals on a piece of paper. Child practices cutting along the lines to cut out the picture. (See Appendix A, pp. 197-202, for sample cutting handouts.)

- Snipping paper: Therapist holds a 1-inch strip of paper and allows the child to make snips in the paper (for lower-level children).

- Child performs resistive cutting activities
  - Child cuts strong Theraputty.
  - Child cuts thick paper.
  - Child cuts several papers at once.

- Craft scissors: Child uses craft scissors to cut paper (craft scissors are more difficult to cut with than regular scissors).

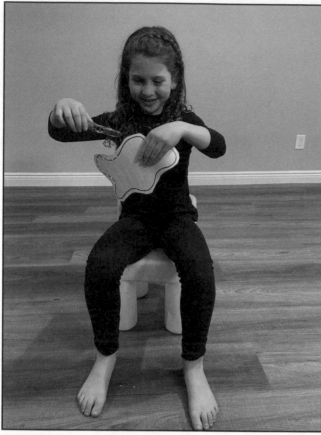

Figure 16-6.

Pressing

- Stapling: Child helps to staple booklets of paper together.
- Hole punching: Therapist draws a line or a shape onto a piece of paper. Child punches holes along the line so that the picture is hole-punched out of the paper (Figure 16-6).

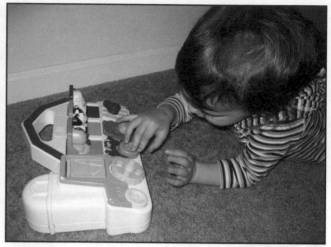

Figure 16-7.

- Child pops bubbles on Bubble Wrap, grabbing bubbles with whole fist.
- Child presses down on pop-up toys (Figure 16-7).

Commercially Available Products

- Bug-Out-Bob
- Mr. Potato Head
- Smart Snacks Sorting Shapes Cupcakes

Handwriting

Handwriting concerns are a primary impetus for an occupational therapy referral in the school-based setting (Reisman, 1991). There is a notable increase in the number of children being referred for school-based occupational therapy due to handwriting deficits (Oliver, 1990). Some studies have shown that 10% to 20% of elementary school students have difficulty with handwriting (Alston & Taylor, 1987). Additionally, there is a significant amount of time dedicated to paper and pencil writing tasks within the classroom (Diekema et al., 1998).

Handwriting interventions can yield significant improvements in various components of overall penmanship skills and legibility (Case-Smith, 2001). In this chapter, various techniques will be introduced in order to promote proper position of the fingers and wrist during writing and proper pencil grasp.

Wrist extension is crucial during writing in order to allow for distal finger movements. In order for the wrist to be in an optimal position, wrist flexors and extensors must work antagonistically and allow proper cocontraction to provide control of the wrist (Benbow, 1997). Various vertical surface writing activities are provided in this chapter as this helps facilitate wrist extension.

Lastly, various pangrams (sentences containing all 26 letters of the alphabet) and sentences including multiple "fall letters" (g, j, p, q, y) are provided in this chapter to enable practice of targeted handwriting skills and letters of focus.

Please refer to Chapter 15 for activities to strengthen the pincer grasp which also can affect proper pencil grasp.

HANDWRITING GAMES

- Rainbow tracing: Child writes the same letter over original template on paper in various colors of the rainbow in order to continually form the same letter.

- Sandpaper writing: Child writes or traces words on regular paper with sandpaper placed underneath the paper to provide proprioceptive input during writing activity.

- Cardboard tracing: Therapist pokes holes in cardboard in the shape of a specific letter. Child then traces over the bumps to form letter (Figures 17-1 and 17-2).

- Child writes letters with small or broken crayons. This will prevent fisting of writing utensil.

- Child uses vibrating pen to trace or write letters.

Danto, A. H., & Pruzansky, M. *1001 Pediatric Treatment Activities:*
Creative Ideas for Therapy Sessions, Third Edition (pp. 103-108).
© 2023 SLACK Incorporated.

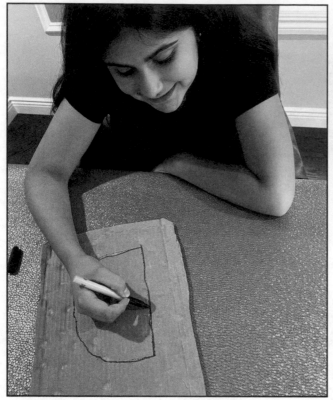

Figure 17-1.

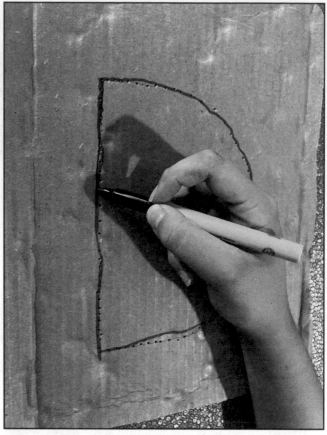

Figure 17-2.

- Therapist and child take turns tracing various letters in each other's palm without looking. Child then has to guess the letter that was traced.

- Air tracing: Child writes letter in the air with extended index finger.

- Foot writing: Child dips toe or foot in paint and then writes a letter on a large paper placed on the floor.

- Sandbox writing: Child writes or traces letters in a sandbox.

- Window writing: Child uses special washable window markers to write letters or words on windows.

- Play-Doh writing
  ○ Child writes letters on flattened piece of Play-Doh.
  ○ Child forms letters out of skinny rolled pieces of Play-Doh.

ACTIVITIES TO PROMOTE DISTAL FINGER MOVEMENTS

- Child colors in small quarter-inch circles of various colors, matching color to the circle (Figures 17-3 and 17-4).

- Child makes a tiny "x" inside small circles all over paper (Figures 17-5 and 17-6).

- Child traces small circles in designated area (Figure 17-7).

- Child traces circle inside paper protector placed on construction paper (Figure 17-8).

- Child traces small lines of varying patterns inside small box on a paper (Figure 17-9).

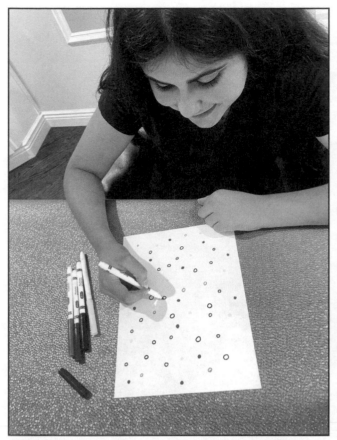

Figure 17-3.

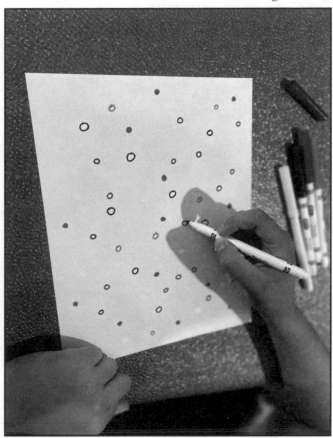

Figure 17-4.

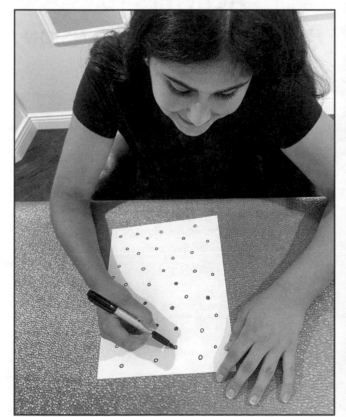

Figure 17-5.

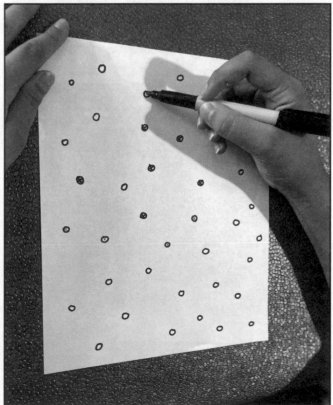

Figure 17-6.

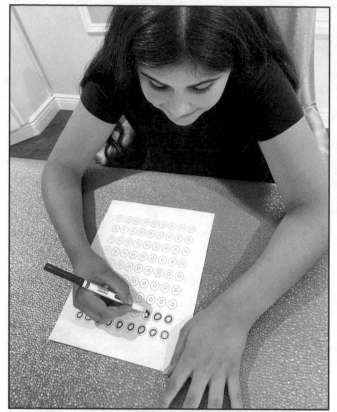

Figure 17-7.

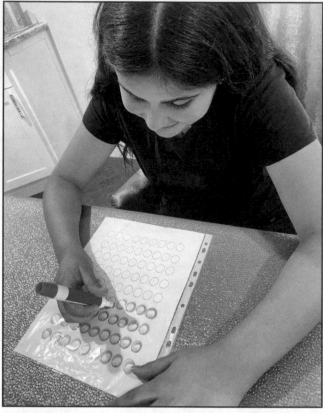

Figure 17-8.

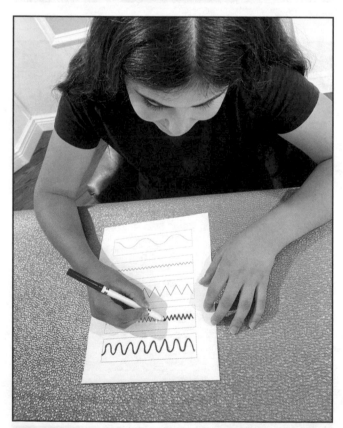

Figure 17-9.

Activities to Promote Wrist Extension

- Have child practice writing with the HandiWriter Handwriting Tool (Figure 17-10).

- Writing on vertical surfaces
  - Child writes on slant board.
  - Therapist places clip board on large binder to simulate slant board for writing.
  - Therapist tapes piece of paper to the wall and child writes on paper.
  - Child writes on whiteboard or chalkboard on the wall.
  - Child writes on a Magna Doodle placed on vertical surface.
  - Child traces over letters with wet sponge or paper towel.

PENCIL GRIPS

Different types of pencil grips address a variety of underlying pencil grasp deficits. Below is a list of various pencil grips that can be purchased:

- DMFLY Pencil Grip
- Crossover Grip
- Writing Claw
- Stetro Pencil Grip
- Geddes Kushy Pencil Grip
- Pencil Grip Jumbo
- Bumpy Grip
- Soft Cushion Pencil Grip
- Foam Grip
- Triangle Pencil Grip

PANGRAMS

The following is a list of pangrams compiled from various websites (Wikipedia, 2020; The Word Play Website, 2020; Your Dictionary, 2020):

- The quick brown fox jumps over the lazy dog.
- Jived fox nymph grabs quick waltz.
- Glib jocks quiz nymph to vex dwarf.
- Sphinx of black quartz, judge my vow.
- How vexingly quick daft zebras jump!
- The five boxing wizards jump quickly.
- Pack my box with five dozen liquor jugs.
- We promptly judged antique ivory buckles for the next prize.
- How razorback jumping frogs can level six piqued gymnasts.
- Sixty zippers were quickly picked from the woven jute bag.
- Crazy Fredrick bought many very exquisite opal jewels.
- Jump by vow of quick, lazy strength in Oxford.
- Quick zephyrs blow, vexing daft Jim.
- Waltz, nymph, for quick jigs vex bud.
- Jackdaws love my big sphinx of quartz.
- Two driven jocks help fax my big quiz.

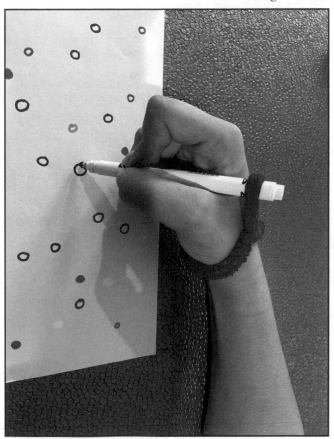

Figure 17-10.

- The jay, pig, fox, zebra, and my wolves quack!
- Sympathizing would fix Quaker objectives.
- A wizard's job is to vex chumps quickly in fog.
- Watch "Jeopardy!", Alex Trebeck's fun TV quiz game.
- By Jove, my quick study of lexicography won a prize!
- Waxy and quivering, jocks fumble the pizza.

The following is a list of sentences with fall letters (g, j, p, q, y):

These sentences include letters that fall below the line and are intended to help work on horizontal alignment awareness.

- The girl picked a green gummy and jelly bean.
- The gift wrap paper was pink and purple.
- The quick piggy played in the muddy pig pen.
- The queen quickly picked a pretty quilt.
- The girl is quietly jumping by herself.
- I lost my key in the gooey plaster.

- Why are you going to be by yourself?
- Peter Piper picked a peck of pickled peppers.
- In gym class the girls were galloping quickly.
- He gives her a shiny penny today.
- I hope you have a happy and joyous birthday.
- The young boy keeps hopping, skipping and playing.
- I suggest you pick apart the wrapping paper before opening the packaged present.
- I'm going on a quick jog with grandma in the pretty park.
- The jester spilled juice on the queen's quilt.
- The funny hippo splashed in the muddy pond.
- The jaguar and puma leaped across the jungle at night.
- The pony hopped and galloped on the foggy day.
- The baby girl plays with her piggy, froggy, and puppy toys.
- She prepped for her quiz every night.
- I'm painting a picture of a penguin gobbling apples and pizza.
- The pampered girl is polishing her nails while wearing pajamas.
- The baby is petting my pet puppy.
- The soapy sponge dripped on the floor and needs to be mopped up.
- We jingled bells, did a jiggy dance, and jumped all night long.
- I prepared yummy popcorn for the party.
- The baby green giant playfully punched and wiggled around.
- We must pick green peas as a healthy and yummy snack.
- It is quite peculiar to pick a purple poncho in the pouring rain.

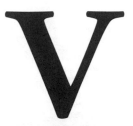

Body Strengthening and Stabilizing

Postural control and stability create the base of support for the rest of the body. There is a significant correlation between decreased core strength and difficulties with dynamic balance (Salar et al., 2014).

This section addresses the various components of body strength and stability. The topics discussed include core-strengthening activities, balance activities, and activities to help improve shoulder and arm stability.

Core-Strengthening Activities

The term *core musculature* refers to the transverse abdominis, internal obliques, pelvic floor, and multifidus muscles (Jeffreys, 2002). Decreased core strength can cause postural insecurity. Ayres (1979) associates postural insecurity with decreased postural mechanisms. Decreased core strength can also result in deficits in fine motor control as well (Shumway-Cook & Woollacott, 1995). Core strength should be one of the first areas addressed in dealing with any fine or gross motor deficit. In this chapter, various core-strengthening exercises are provided to help establish a strong foundation on which to build further skills.

It is important that when performing activities with infants, small children, and developmentally delayed children, the therapist should be skilled in proper handling techniques in order to safely and effectively implement the chosen activity. To become familiar with these handling techniques, the therapist should contact a trained pediatric occupational or physical therapist familiar with the specific population of interest.

CORE-STRENGTHENING ACTIVITIES

Abdominal Exercises

- Modified sit-up: Place child on back on the floor or soft surface. Pull child's hands gently at the same time and let child use abdominal muscles to pull self to upright, seated position (developmental age of 4 to 6 months; Figure 18-1)

- "Row, Row, Row Your Boat" game: In this game, child sits on the floor, facing either therapist or another child, each holding onto one end of a jump rope (position I) or onto each other's wrists (position II). As both sing the song, one person leans back as the other leans forward and then the opposite.

  ○ Position I (Figure 18-2).

  ○ Position II (Figure 18-3).

- Sit-ups and crunches: Child performs sit-ups and crunches on the floor. Therapist performs the same exercises with child to help keep child motivated (developmental age of 6 years and up).

Danto, A. H., & Pruzansky, M. *1001 Pediatric Treatment Activities: Creative Ideas for Therapy Sessions, Third Edition* (pp. 111-120).
© 2023 SLACK Incorporated.

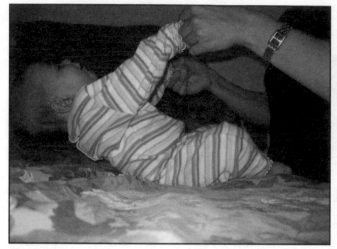

Figure 18-1.

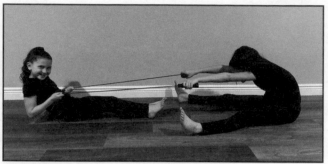

Figure 18-2.

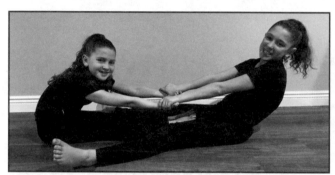

Figure 18-3.

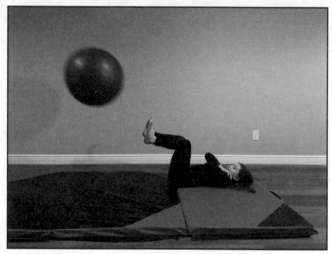

Figure 18-4.

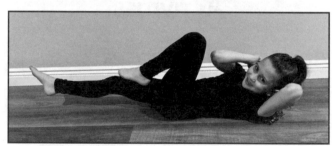

Figure 18-5.

- Feet kick: Child lies supine (on back) on a mat with feet in the air. Therapist throws a large therapy ball toward child's feet. Child kicks ball upward and back toward therapist (Figure 18-4).

- Leg lifts: Child lies flat on floor and raises and lowers legs off the floor (developmental age of 6 years and up).

- Bicycle sit-ups: Child lies on back and brings the right elbow to the left knee, while extending the right leg. Then switches and repeats as tolerated (developmental age of 6 years and up; Figure 18-5).

- Therapist lies on floor opposite child with therapist's feet touching child's feet. Therapist places a small ball between therapist's ankles and passes the ball to child.

Child takes ball between child's ankles and passes ball back to the therapist in same way. This can also be played with two children (Figures 18-6 through 18-8).

- Backward flip: Child lies on back on therapy ball. Child places arms on floor for support behind self. Child then flips body over (Figure 18-9).

Whole-Body Stabilization

- Sitting exercises (developmental age of 6 to 8 months)

   ○ Therapist places the child on lap with the child facing therapist. Therapist holds child's hands and engages child while also lifting up one of child's knees and then the other, shifting child's weight from side to side.

   ○ Weight shifting: Therapist places child in sitting position on floor, providing minimal support. Therapist gently tilts child off balance to each side (one at a time) and then forward and backward. Therapist should try to tilt child only slightly so that child is able to regain balance and an upright, seated position independently when possible.

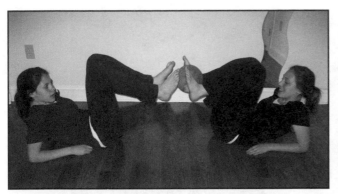

Figure 18-6.

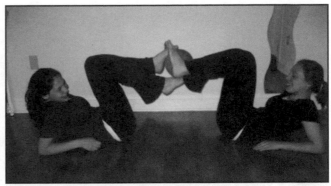

Figure 18-7.

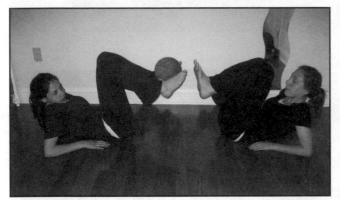

Figure 18-8.

- Therapist places child in sitting position for play and interaction with Boppy pillow around child for support (Figure 18-10).

- Therapist places Hip Helpers (www.hiphelpers.com) on child to provide extra support while sitting. Hip Helpers prevent the child from "W" sitting (or sitting with legs spread wide apart, forming a wide base of support), thus "forcing" child to activate their trunk muscles while sitting.

- Therapist places child in sitting position on floor, providing minimal support as needed. Therapist allows child to stay in this position as tolerated while engaging in playful activities (Figure 18-11).

- While child is sitting, therapist holds a favorite toy, such as a rattle, just above child's head and encourages child to reach for the toy. Therapist should have several different toys on hand so this can be repeated several times in a row.

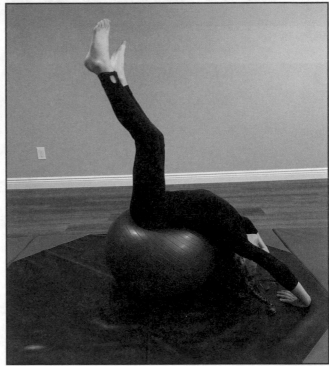

Figure 18-9.

- Therapist can place the toys on all sides of child so that child is required to reach in different directions to acquire the toys.

- Standing exercises (developmental age of 3 to 4 months; Cottrell, 2004, p. 20): Have child practice standing with limited support. Hold child under armpits (Figure 18-12) or by the hands (Figure 18-13), providing minimal support as needed. Place child's feet on a steady surface. Have child practice standing for several seconds at a time as tolerated.

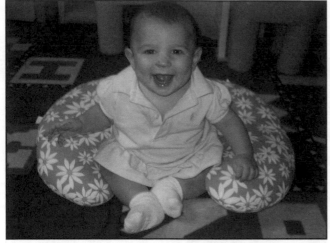

Figure 18-10.

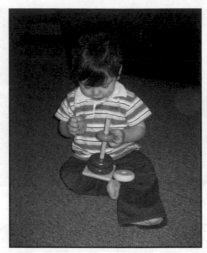

Figure 18-11.

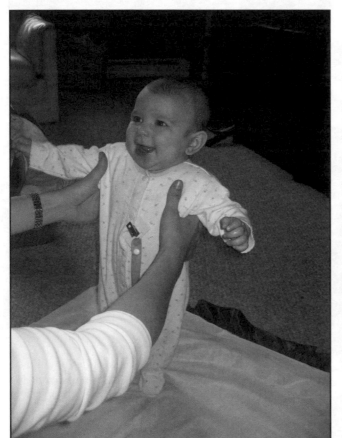

Figure 18-12.

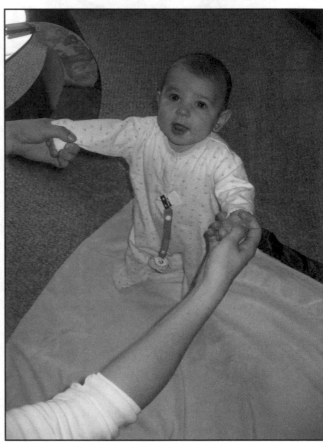

Figure 18-13.

- Kneeling activities: Child performs activities while kneeling on the floor (Figures 18-14 and 18-15). While there are many games that can be played in this position, some ideas include coloring activities, completing puzzles, playing catch, playing a card game on a low stool, and rolling a ring across the floor (do not allow child to lean body against surface to support self when in unstable positions).

- Child slowly walks up a ramp. Therapist makes sure child is standing upright and not using the hands or head to help climb.

- Dizzy Disc: Child spins on the disc without falling off (Figure 18-16).

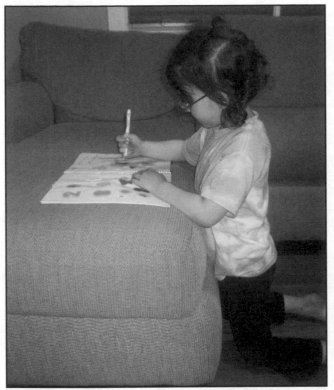

Figure 18-14.

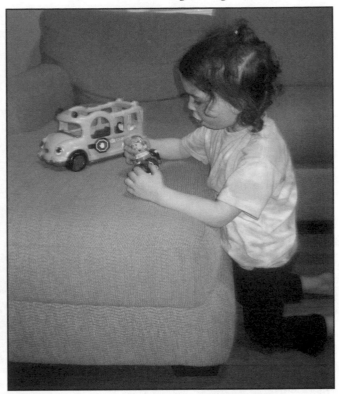

Figure 18-15.

- Child sits on a bolster or peanut ball and reaches for far items placed on both sides. Child then throws the items into a basket (Figure 18-17).

- Couch push-ups: Child lies prone (on the belly) on a couch, perpendicular to the length of the couch, with the upper body off the couch and hands on the floor and then performs push-ups (Figure 18-18). Child can also play a game or do a puzzle in this position.

- Step-ups: Child steps up and down from an object approximately a foot off of the floor. Therapist reminds child to place both arms out to the side when stepping onto and off of the surface to prevent them from compensating by using arm muscles (Figure 18-19).

- Hippity Hop toy: Child bounces across room on a Hippity Hop toy (Figure 18-20; this toy can also be used as part of a relay race).

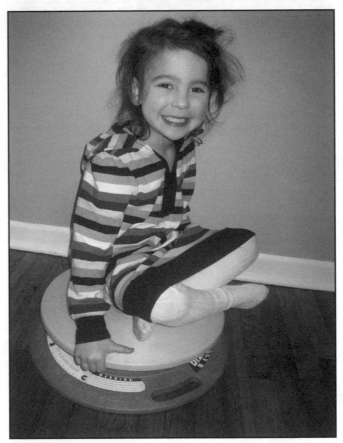

Figure 18-16.

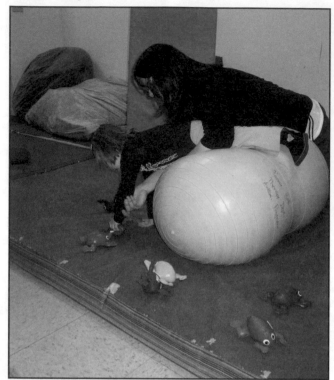

Figure 18-17.

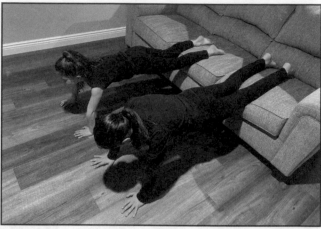

Figure 18-18.

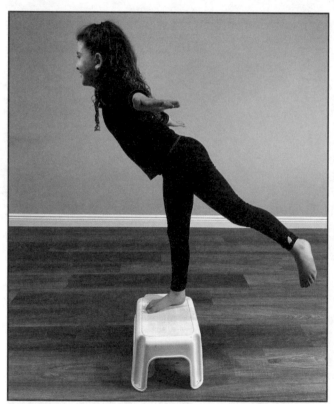

Figure 18-19.

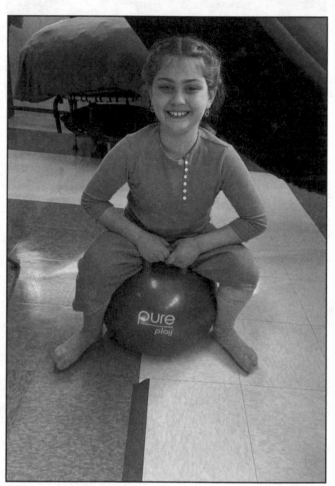

Figure 18-20.

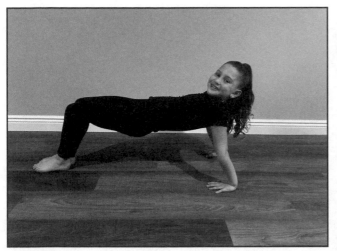

Figure 18-21.

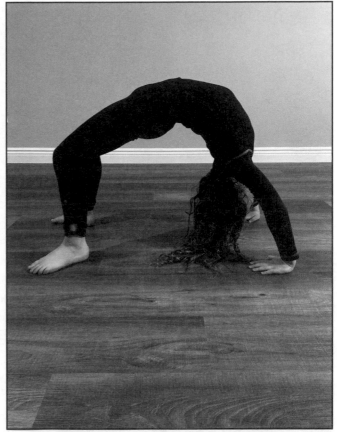

Figure 18-22.

- Crab-walking: Child crab-walks across the room and picks up different objects along the way (Figure 18-21).

- Bridge making: Child lies on back on the floor. Therapist helps child make a bridge. Child then attempts to make a bridge independently (Figures 18-22* and 18-23*; child can also make a bridge over a therapy ball.)

- Limbo: Child walks under a stick in the game of limbo. Therapist should make sure that child leans backward in walking under the stick and not forward or else child will not be using abdominal muscles.

- Pogo stick jumping: Child jumps across room on a pogo stick.

Suspended Equipment Activities

Therapist must make sure that a mat or soft surface is placed under all suspended equipment while in use.

- Therapist wraps child's legs around a T-swing. Child goes upside down and then tries to pull self up (Figure 18-24*).

- Log swing
  - Child straddles log swing and goes back and forth on moving swing without falling off.
  - Child hangs upside-down on swing and holds on for a set count. Child then performs this activity several more times trying to beat own record for time held on (Figure 18-25*; This activity can be made more challenging by reaching for items on floor while hanging upside down).

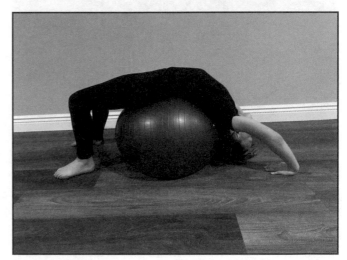

Figure 18-23.

Increased caution should be taken with these activities, especially with children with lax ligaments or any medical conditions that may make them susceptible to dislocations or where head inversions are contraindicated.

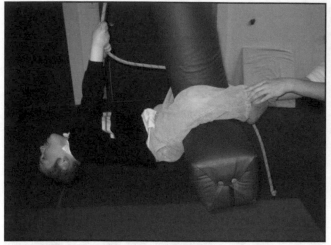

Figure 18-24.

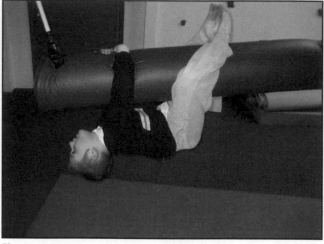

Figure 18-25.

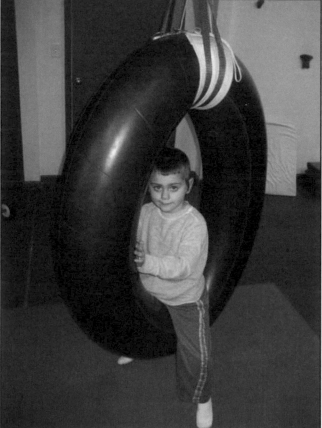

Figure 18-26.

- Tire swing: Child straddles tire. Therapist makes sure child is not leaning forward or backward, rather sitting upright so that the back and belly are not touching the tire. Therapist swings tire back and forth and side to side. Child holds on as long as possible (Figure 18-26).
- Child hangs upside down on a trapeze bar and pulls self up (Figure 18-27*).
- Lycra swing: Child climbs up a long Lycra swing to the top and then slides down.

Therapy Ball Activities

- Child holds therapy ball against wall only with body (no hands). Child plants feet on floor and creates a bouncing momentum against the ball.
- Child holds a large therapy ball against the wall only with body and then slightly moves ball back and forth along the wall using their chest and stomach without using hands (Figure 18-28).
- Therapist places child in sitting position on therapy ball. While holding onto child, therapist rolls ball forward and backward and from side to side while engaging the child.

*Increased caution should be taken with these activities, especially with children with lax ligaments or any medical conditions that may make them susceptible to dislocations or where head inversions are contraindicated.

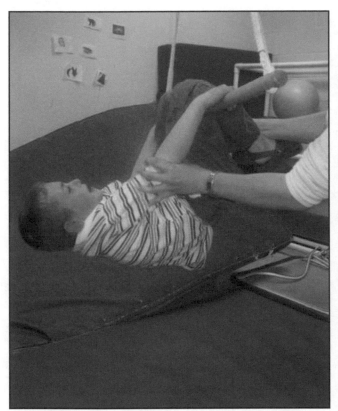

Figure 18-27.

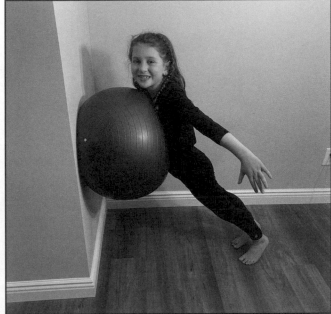

Figure 18-28.

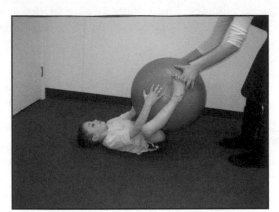

Figure 18-29.

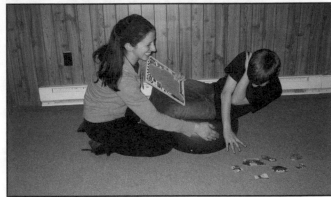

Figure 18-30.

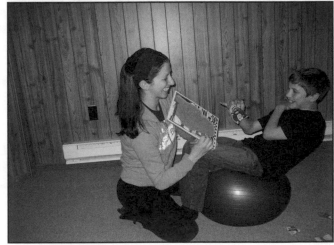

Figure 18-31.

- Child lies on back on the floor and holds therapy ball with both feet and hands. Therapist tries to gently pry ball away from child while child tries to hold onto ball (Figure 18-29).

- Puzzle–ball sit-ups: Therapist scatters puzzle pieces around a therapy ball. Child sits on therapy ball and reaches for puzzle pieces placed behind or on the side of the ball. Child then performs a sit-up to put the piece into the puzzle frame (Figures 18-30 and 18-31).

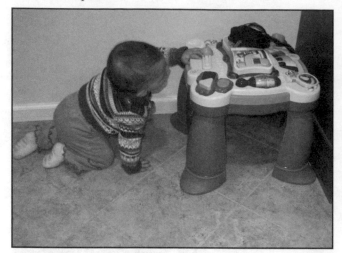

Figure 18-32.

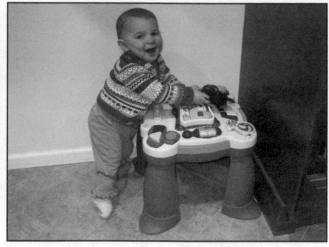

Figure 18-33.

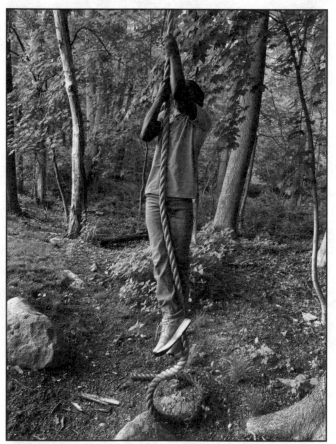

Figure 18-34.

Climbing

- Climbing up furniture: Therapist brings child near a chair, couch, or small table. Therapist places a desired toy on the surface and encourages/assists child, as minimally as possible, to transition from either sitting or quadruped to standing while holding onto couch or chair to reach for toy (Figures 18-32 and 18-33).

- Ladder climbing: Child climbs up a ladder, net, or rope in the therapy area or outside on playground (Figure 18-34).

- Rock wall games

  ○ Child climbs up wall.

  ○ Child climbs up rock wall, using only one rock of a specific color.

  ○ Therapist scatters rings on the top and along rock wall. Child climbs across rock wall, picks up rings, and throws them into a basket.

19

Balance Activities

Balance is required for smooth and coordinated movement. There is a correlation between decreased balance and adverse effects on fine motor skills (Burnett et al., 2011). Some children will have a postural disorder that affects balance and may include poor righting and equilibrium reactions, poor weight shifting and difficulty with trunk rotation (Miller et al., 2007).

There is various literature on the efficacy of balance training programs and treatments geared at improving standing and dynamic balance (Shumway-Cook et al., 2003). Balance training interventions have also shown improvements in postural control with people with autism spectrum disorder (Cheldavi et al., 2014). Specifically, postural control can be strengthened through balance training activities (Granacher et al., 2010). Engaging in core strength exercises is another way to improve balance (Granacher et al., 2013).

Specifically, the balance activities included in this chapter are those that require the child to be on one foot or to maintain balance on unstable surfaces. A child lives in a dynamic environment. For example, they will need to learn to walk on uneven sidewalks, up and down curbs, and over bumps on a grassy surface. A child who is able to maintain balance only on stable and static surfaces would face serious difficulties in real world situations. Activities to strengthen protective reactions are included as well. Protective reactions occur in the frontward and backward as well as in the lateral plane of movement. A protective reaction occurs when one is falling and "catches" oneself by stretching out one's arms in the direction of the fall. These reactions also occur in forward, backward, and lateral directions (Case-Smith, 2001).

Danto, A. H., & Pruzansky, M. *1001 Pediatric Treatment Activities:*
Creative Ideas for Therapy Sessions, Third Edition (pp. 121-127).
© 2023 SLACK Incorporated.

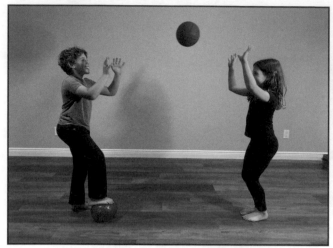

Figure 19-1.

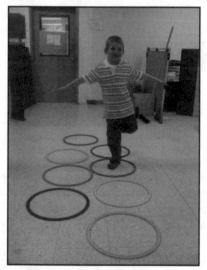

Figure 19-3.

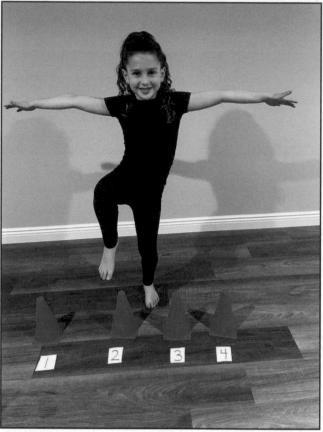

Figure 19-2.

BALANCE ACTIVITIES

All activities in this chapter must be done with close adult supervision, especially with children who have poor balance skills.

One-Foot Activities

- Child maintains balance on one foot for X seconds and then alternates to other for X seconds. (Amount of time should be determined by treating therapist.)

- Child stands on one foot with other foot resting on a ball. Therapist stabilizes the ball if needed. To make activity more challenging, child performs an activity while on one foot—for example, while playing catch, clapping hands, etc. (Figure 19-1).

- Tapping cones with one foot: Child stands on one foot. Therapist places numbered (or colored) cones on floor approximately a foot away from child. Therapist calls out a number (or color) and child taps corresponding cone while maintaining balance (Figure 19-2).

- Hopping activities

  o Child hops into rings placed on floor and freezes (Figure 19-3).

  o Child hops over bumpy balance board sections (Figure 19-4).

  o Child hops in place.

  o Therapist places laminated letters all around the floor. Child hops over the letters of child's name.

  o Therapist places a rope on floor and tapes it down on both ends. Child hops over the rope and back (Figure 19-5).

  o Therapist places a rope on floor and tapes it down on both ends. Starting from one end of the rope, child hops over the rope, alternating landing on each side of the rope, making their way along the length of the rope while hopping, until they reach the other end.

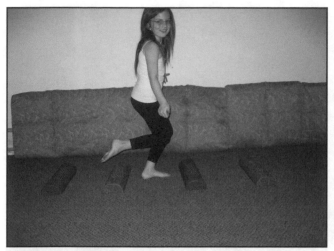

Figure 19-4.

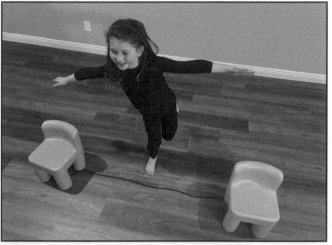

Figure 19-5.

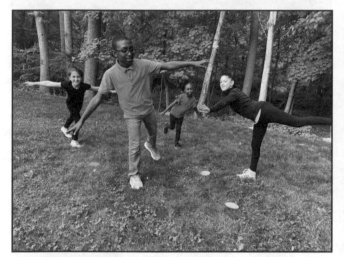

Figure 19-6.

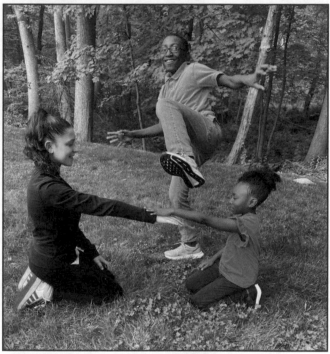

- Balance on it: Therapist calls out a body part. Child balances on that body part. Some examples include right foot, left foot, both knees, one knee, both hands, etc. (Figure 19-6).

- Human maze: Children lock arms to create a human obstacle course. Another child will have to balance and climb over the human maze (Figure 19-7).

- Child passes ball under leg to another child. Other child receives ball and repeats activity to pass ball back (Figures 19-8 and 19-9).

Standing/Walking on Unstable Surfaces

- Balance-board activities
  - Child steps on/off balance board.
  - Child turns around in a 360-degree circle.
  - Child plays catch with therapist.

Figure 19-7.

  - Child pops bubbles in air (Figure 19-10).
  - Child reaches across midline for items in the air (Figure 19-11).
  - Child plays basketball (Figure 19-12).
  - Child throws a ball against a wall and catches it (Figure 19-13).
  - Child places bean bag on head and balances it while on balance board.
- Balance beam activities
  - Child walks across balance beam.
  - Child picks up items from the floor and throws them into target (Figure 19-14).

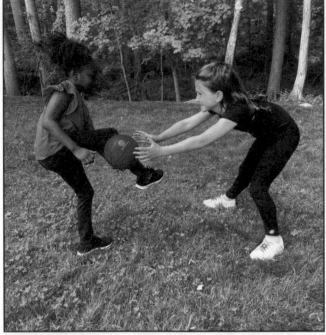

Figure 19-8.

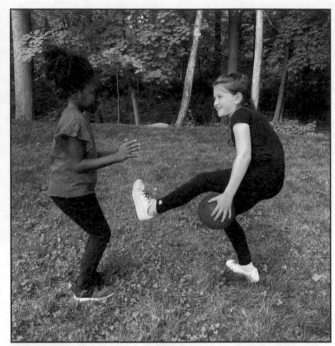

Figure 19-9.

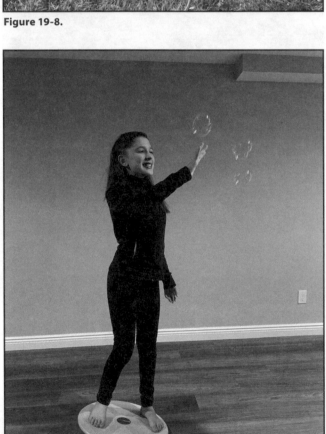

Figure 19-10.

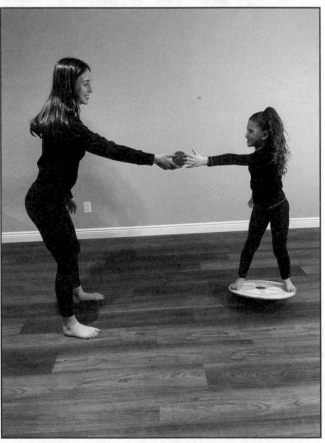

Figure 19-11.

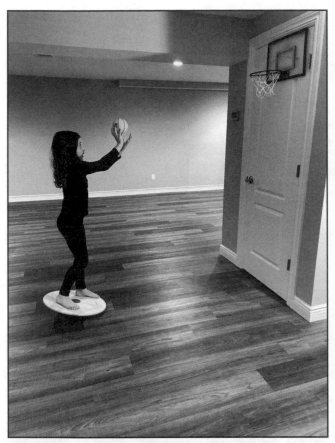

Figure 19-12.

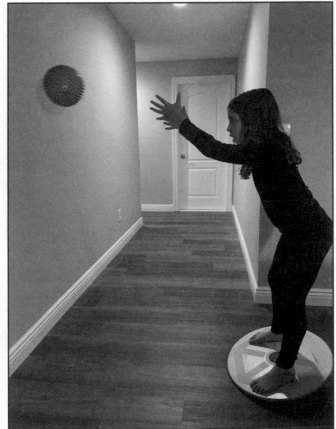

Figure 19-13.

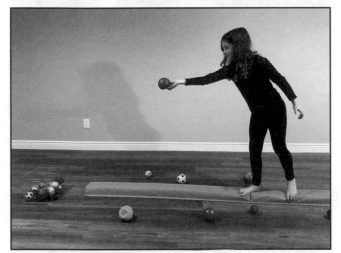

Figure 19-14.

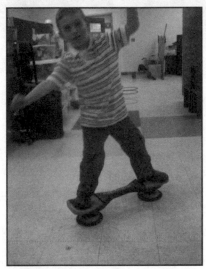

Figure 19-15.

- ○ Child walks across balance beam while holding an object in both hands.
- ○ Child plays catch on balance beam.
- ○ Child stands still, maintaining standing balance.
- Inflatable air disc: Child maintains balance with both feet placed on inflatable disc.

- ○ This activity can be downgraded by allowing child's toes to slide slightly forward and make contact with the floor (as opposed to being completely grounded on the air disc).
- Woggler: Child walks across the room on a Woggler (Figure 19-15).

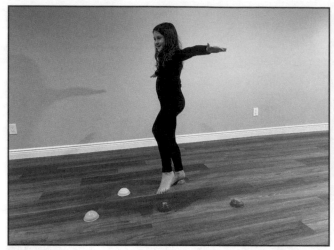

Figure 19-16.

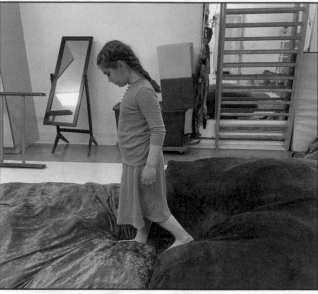

Figure 19-17.

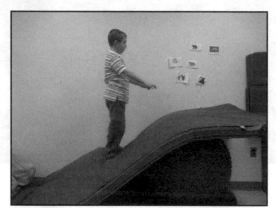

Figure 19-18.

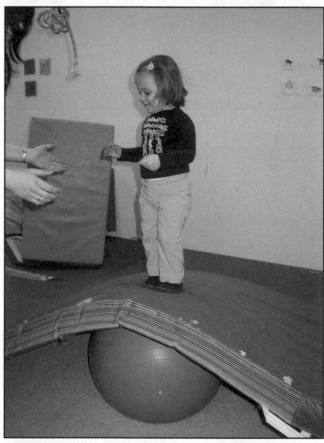

Figure 19-19.

- Stepping stones: Child walks onto a specific colored or numbered stone (Figure 19-16).

- Child walks on beanbags or other uneven surfaces (Figure 19-17).

- Therapist places a therapy ball under a mat/ramp. Child walks up the mat/ramp (Figure 19-18).

- Therapist places therapy ball under mat. Child "surfs" by balancing on moving mat and standing in one place (Figure 19-19).

- Therapist places log swing on floor. Child walks across it without falling off. (Therapist may need to stabilize swing on the floor so it does not move around too much when the child is walking across it.)

- Curb-walking: Child walks outside along the sidewalk curb.

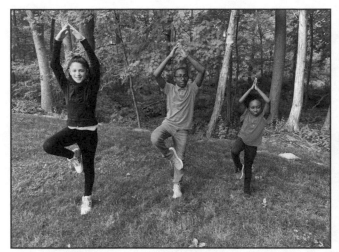

Figure 19-20.

- Walking on straight line: Child walks along a straight piece of long tape placed on the floor.
- Stair climbing

Therapist must guard child while performing these activities and be done with close supervision.

  ○ Child walks up and down stairs without using railing.
  ○ Child walks backward up stairs and then down again.

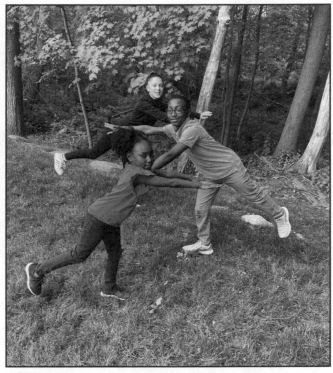

Figure 19-21.

Alternative Forms of Exercise

- Karate
- Pilates
- Yoga (Figures 19-20 and 19-21)

Upper Arm Strengthening and Stabilization

Upper arm strength and stability are essential to the functional use of the hands. It is a long-standing belief among physical and occupational therapists that proximal control is a prerequisite for distal arm functioning (Tudor, 1981). Children with poor upper arm strength and stability frequently have difficulty performing tasks with their hands. Proximal stability of the shoulder and surrounding musculature is necessary for distal arm control and proper use of the hand (Benbow, 1995).

This chapter provides a variety of activities to help strengthen and stabilize the arm and shoulder area. Weight-bearing activities can often provide stability to the shoulder joint. This chapter also includes activities that can be performed on a vertical surface, which can result in improved use of the thumb (Benbow, 1995).

UPPER ARM STRENGTHENING AND STABILIZATION

Bearing Weight Through the Hands

- Place child in prone weight-bearing position so that child bears weight through forearms or hands.

- Lie on floor next to child, slightly higher than eye level. Alternatively, place child in prone position on a bed surface to make it easier for adult to be at child's eye level (Figure 20-1).

- Place child on Boppy pillow or elevated surface in order to improve tolerance toward being in a prone position (developmental age 4 to 6 months; Figure 20-2).

- Increase supervised "tummy time" activities for young children (developmental age 4 to 6 months).

  ○ Therapist lies at slight angle on floor, couch, or bed and places child on stomach/chest area in prone position (Figure 20-3).

Danto, A. H., & Pruzansky, M. *1001 Pediatric Treatment Activities: Creative Ideas for Therapy Sessions, Third Edition* (pp. 129-138).
© 2023 SLACK Incorporated.

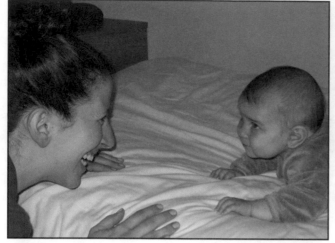

Figure 20-1.

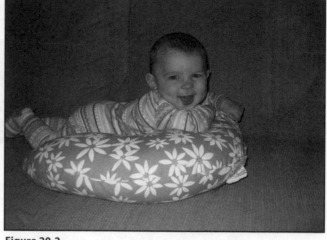

Figure 20-2.

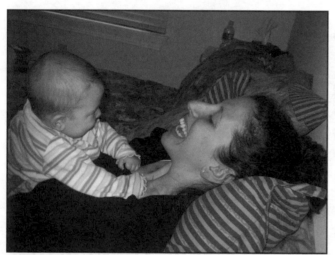

Figure 20-3.

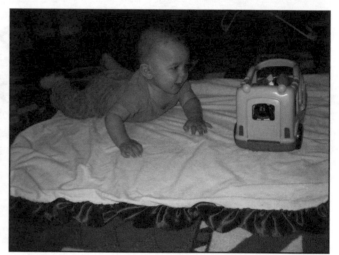

Figure 20-4.

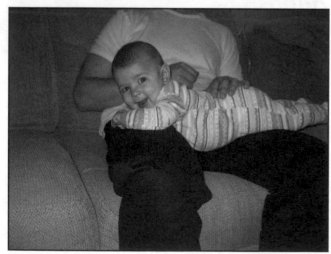

Figure 20-5.

- ○ Place a thin soft blanket on floor and place a toy in front of child on belly (Figure 20-4).
- ○ Place child on stomach in front of a mirror.
- ○ Place child on stomach over therapist's lap (Figure 20-5).
- ○ Hold child horizontally in air, weight bearing on adult's forearm (Figure 20-6).
- Place child in quadruped position
  - ○ Have child maintain stationary position.
  - ○ Have child reach for items from this position (Figure 20-7).
  - ○ Have child go through crawling movements from this position with the therapist facilitating the movement.

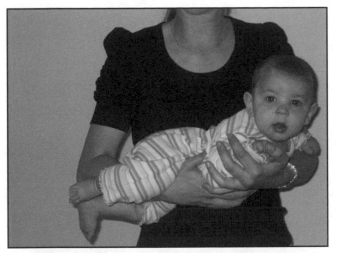

Figure 20-6.

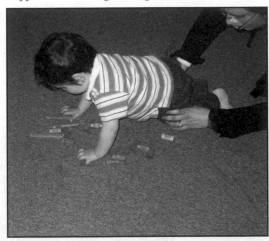

Figure 20-7.

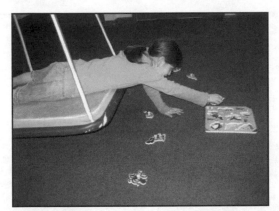

Figure 20-8.

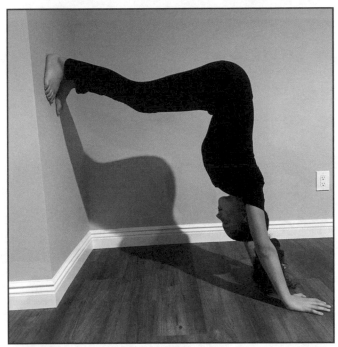

Figure 20-9.

- Child lies in prone position (on the belly) on a platform swing or a net swing a few inches off floor. Child leans over the edge so the chest is not on the swing, but rather off the edge. Therapist spreads out objects all around and under the swing. Child walks on hands to objects, picks them up, and throws them into a container, or performs another task with them (Figure 20-8).

- Child lies prone (on belly) on a scooter board. Child holds onto a bungee cord or jump rope while being pulled by therapist.

- Child lies prone on a scooter board and propels self around the room in order to reach and pick up objects. For example, child picks up scattered bean bags or Koosh balls all over the floor and then places them into a bucket.

- Child walks feet up the wall while weight bearing through the hands on a mat (Figure 20-9).

- Crab-walking: Child walks in a supine (on back) position on hands and feet making sure that no other parts of the body are touching the floor (Figure 20-10).

- Wheelbarrow walking
  - Child maintains a stationary wheelbarrow position.
  - Child reaches for toys in this position.
  - Child walks on hands with legs being held up in the air (Figure 20-11). This activity can be graded by the distance walked and where the therapist places support when holding the child's legs. It is most physically challenging for the child when being held around the ankles. The closer to the hip the support is provided, the easier the activity for the child.

- Wheelbarrow-walking races (Figure 20-12).

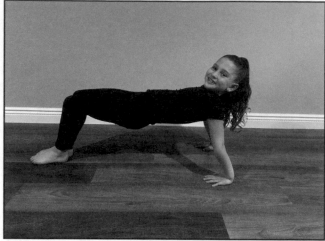

Figure 20-10.

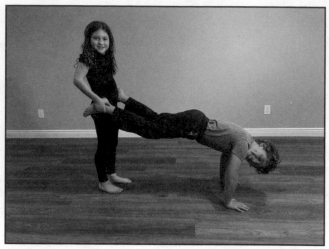

Figure 20-11.

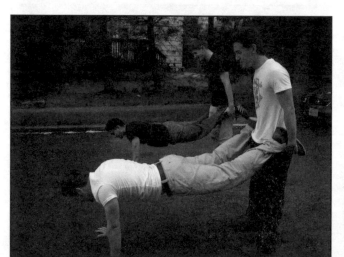

Figure 20-12.

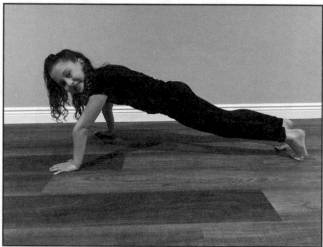

Figure 20-13.

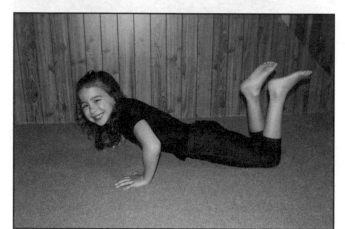

Figure 20-14.

- Push-ups: Child performs different push-ups.
  - Regular floor push-ups (Figure 20-13).
  - Half push-ups with knees touching floor (Figure 20-14).

- Wall push-ups (Figure 20-15).
  - Couch push-ups: Child lies on a couch on belly, hanging over the edge. Child places arms on the floor and pushes off the floor keeping lower body on the couch (Figure 20-16).
  - Chair push-ups: Child sits on a chair, grabs each side of the chair with hands, locks elbows, pushes down, all while keeping bottom seated on chair (Figure 20-17).
- Child leans over the edge of a solid stable surface, so that the chest is not supported by the surface. Therapist spreads puzzle pieces around the floor within arm's length. Child reaches for pieces and completes the puzzle (Figure 20-18).
- Child is placed prone on therapy ball while bearing weight through the arms. Child performs push-ups in this position (Figures 20-19 and 20-20).

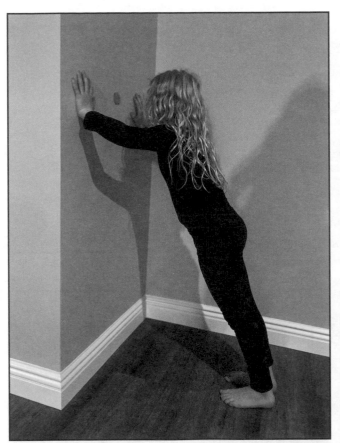

Figure 20-15.

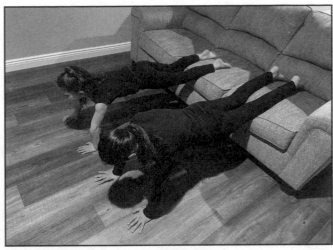

Figure 20-16.

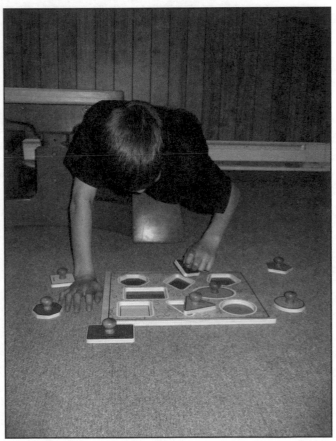

Figure 20-18.

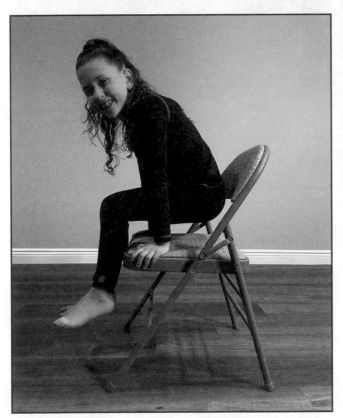

Figure 20-17.

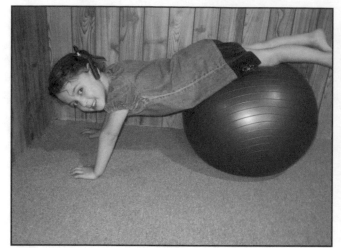

Figure 20-19.

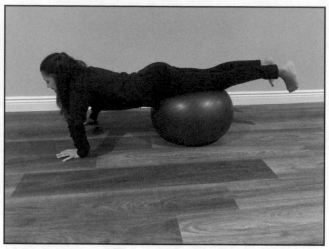

Figure 20-20.

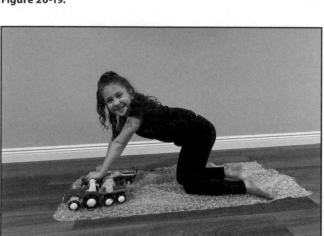

Figure 20-21.

- Bubble Wrap popping: Therapist places sheet of Bubble Wrap on floor in a line. Child takes rolling truck or car and places it on top of Bubble Wrap paper and presses down on rolling truck as it is rolled over the line of Bubble Wrap (Figure 20-21).

Using Vertical Surfaces

The following activities work best on shoulder stabilization when the arm is in a position at and above shoulder level (90 degrees of shoulder flexion).

- Vertical surface writing
  - Child colors on an easel.
  - Child writes on a chalkboard.
  - Child traces letters on a whiteboard.

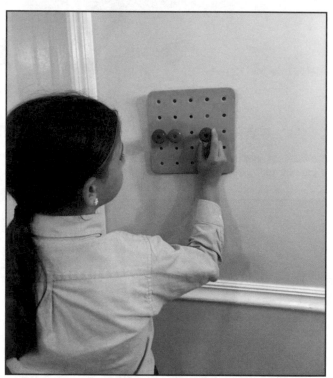

Figure 20-22.

  - Child completes writing sheets on a slantboard.
  - Child colors piece of paper taped onto the wall. (Child can color, paint, or write on this surface.)
- Child cleans off the chalkboard with an eraser or wet paper towel.
- Child pushes pegs into a peg board on vertical surface (Figure 20-22).
- Child places magnets on a vertical surface.

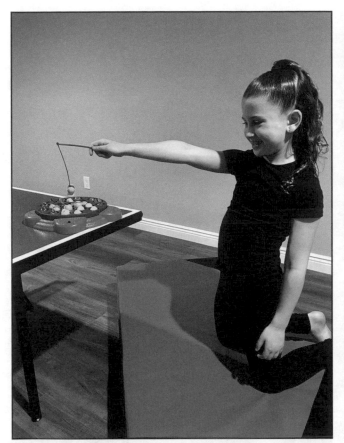

Figure 20-23.

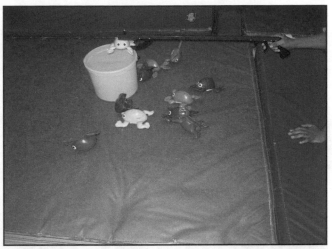

Figure 20-24.

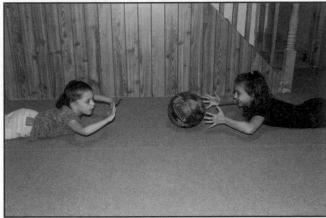

Figure 20-26.

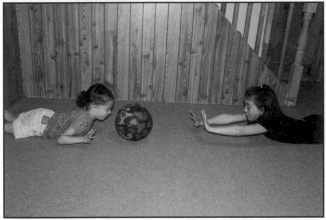

Figure 20-25.

Stabilizing the Shoulder Against Gravity

The following activities provided work best on shoulder stabilization when the arm is in a position at and above shoulder level (90 degrees of shoulder flexion).

- Child swings a jump rope.
- Child holds arms up in the air for X number of seconds. (Amount of time should be determined by treating therapist.)
- Child plays a game with magnetic fishing rods. Child uses the rod to lift up the fish when magnets connect (Figure 20-23).
- Child builds a tower with blocks.
- Child lies prone on a platform swing. Child uses a reacher to pick up scattered beanbags/toys and places them into a bucket (Figure 20-24). To upgrade or downgrade this activity, therapist can put the bucket at different heights and distances away from child.
- Child lies prone on floor and faces another child or therapist lying on belly. Both children pass ball by rolling it on the floor back and forth between them (Figures 20-25 and 20-26).

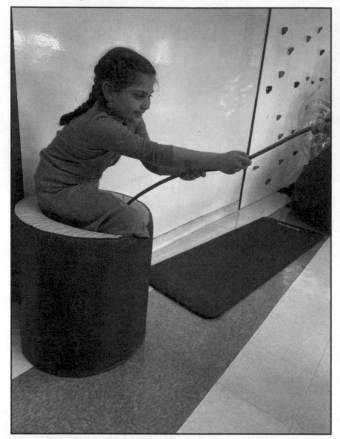

Figure 20-27.

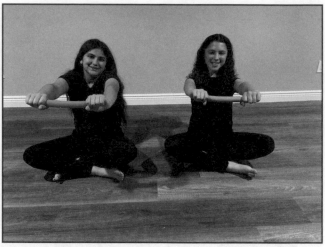

Figure 20-28.

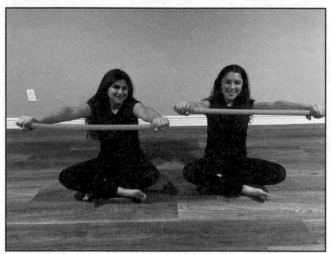

Figure 20-29.

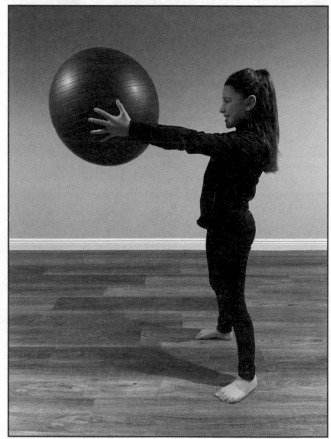

Figure 20-30.

Resistive Activities

- Child sits in a storage bin or barrel and pulls self out by climbing a rope that is being pulled tightly by therapist (Figure 20-27).

- Child pulls apart Rapper Snappers or Therabands with arms straight out in front (Figures 20-28 and 20-29).

- Child places a mid-sized therapy ball between hands with arms straight out in front of body and walks across the room holding the ball (Figure 20-30). Use a smaller ball if this is too challenging.

- Child climbs up a ladder.

- Child swings on a trapeze bar.

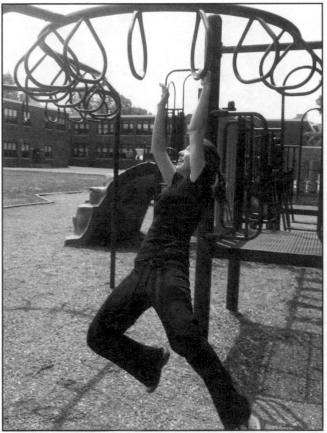

Figure 20-31.

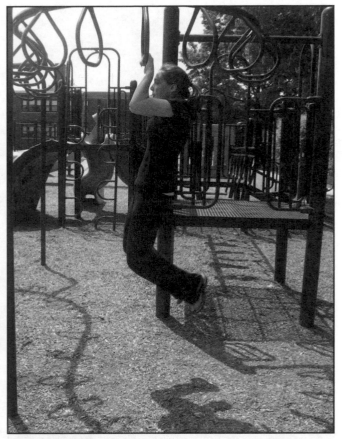

Figure 20-32.

- Child swings across monkey bars in the playground (Figure 20-31).

- Child hangs on monkey bar in place (Figure 20-32).

- Theraband exercises
  - Child holds Theraband out in front of the body with both hands, pulls apart, holds, and repeats as tolerated (Figure 20-33).
  - Child places Theraband behind the back with the Theraband wrapped around so child can grab it with each hand on both sides. Child straightens arms out to the side and holds. Repeat as tolerated (Figure 20-34).

- Hula Hoop pulling: Therapist places child on a swing or a scooter while child holds onto a Hula Hoop. Therapist holds onto the other end of the hoop and pulls child around.

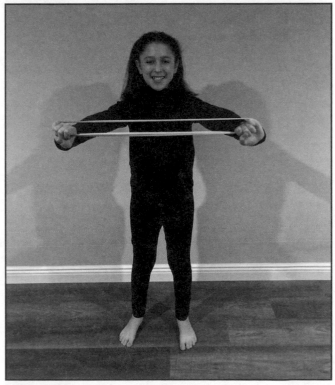

Figure 20-33.

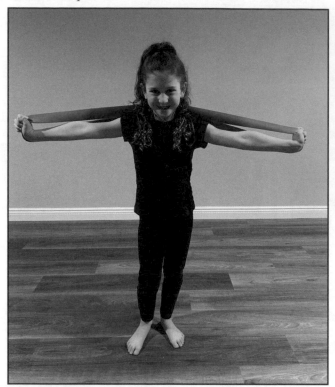

Figure 20-34.

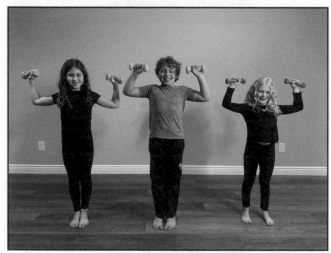

Figure 20-36.

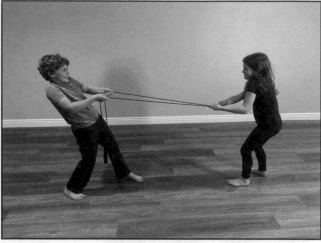

Figure 20-35.

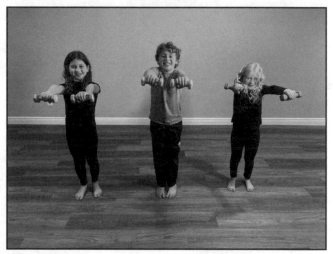

Figure 20-37.

Commercially Available Products

- Don't Spill the Beans
- Fantacolor Junior
- Jenga
- Lite Brite
- Magnet Express
- Melissa & Doug Magnetic Puzzles
- Zoom Ball

- Tug-of-war: This game can be played between child and therapist or between two children. This game should be closely supervised for safety concerns (Figure 20-35).

- Lifting weights: In a standing position, child holds weight in each hand at shoulder height with flexed elbows (Figure 20-36). Child fully extends arms and maintains shoulder flexion at 90 degrees (Figure 20-37). Repeat a certain number of times (number of repetitions should be determined by treating therapist).

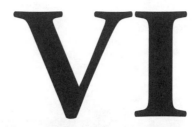

Cognitive and Higher-Level Skill Building

Cognitive skills and executive functioning are critical for complex child behavior (Biederman et al., 2004). Studies of various diseases show the significance of executive functioning and how deficits in executive functioning will result in large functional impairments (Chen et al., 1998).

Included in this section are activities that will help to improve overall organizational skills related to cognition and executive functioning. As described by Zeigler-Dendy (2002), components of executive functioning that affect school performance include the following:

- Working memory and recall (holding facts in mind while manipulating information, accessing facts stored in long-term memory).
- Activation, arousal, and effort (getting started, paying attention, finishing work).
- Controlling emotions (ability to tolerate frustration, thinking before acting or speaking).
- Internalizing language (using "self-talk" to control one's behavior and direct future actions).
- Taking an issue apart, analyzing the pieces, and reconstituting and organizing it into new ideas (complex problem solving).

This section addresses specific areas of cognition and higher-level skill building, including increasing attention and improving organizational skills.

21

Increasing Attention

Being able to maintain attention is a prerequisite to engagement and completion of any activity (Ben-Yishay et al., 1987). This chapter discusses three main types of attention: visual attention, sustained attention, and shifted/divided attention. Sustained attention is the ability to maintain attention on a specific point for a considerable length of time. Shifted/divided attention refers to the ability to move attention from one task to another. Many children, especially those with developmental disabilities will demonstrate difficulties with sustained attention to a task (Cardona et al., 2000). When a child is unable to attend or focus, this will often cause difficulties with learning and peer interaction (DeGangi, 1994).

The types of activities suggested in this chapter are those that require continued engagement for a successful outcome. Most activities and games provided require both forms of attention. A therapist working on these skills may downgrade the task by focusing on only one form of attention at a time. It is at the discretion of the treating therapist to upgrade any activity as needed.

Other helpful strategies for increasing attention include the following:

- The therapist should prepare the treatment area before treating a child to avoid having to stop an activity to obtain needed toys or materials.

- It may be helpful to work and play in a tent/tunnel or cubicle to avoid outside distractions.

- When working with a higher-level child, try working or playing with music in background. This can help to strengthen the child's ability to tune out extraneous background noise and focus on the demands at hand. This should be done only with a child who has already mastered the skill of being able to focus in a quiet, distraction-free environment.

- Perform fast-paced activities to help the child stay focused.

- Computer-based learning games and activities are commonly used to help increase attention as they provide continuous and immediate feedback (Cardona et al., 2000).

Danto, A. H., & Pruzansky, M. *1001 Pediatric Treatment Activities:*
Creative Ideas for Therapy Sessions, Third Edition (pp. 141-142).
© 2023 SLACK Incorporated.

ACTIVITIES TO
INCREASE ATTENTION

Visual Attention

- Therapist plays Peek-a-Boo with child.
- Child bounces on a therapy ball or sits on an air disc while playing a game.
- Child visually tracks an object in different planes (choose an object that is desirable to the child).

Higher-Level Attention Building

- Copy a pattern: Child laces beads in a pattern of colors or shapes.
- Child colors lines on a paper in a specific pattern. Child repeats the pattern out loud in a sing-song way as a memory tool.
- ABC wall game: Therapist places the letters A through E on the wall approximately half-an-inch apart in a random order. The letters should be large enough so a child can stand a few feet away from the wall and still see them. Child throws a ball at letter "A" and catches it; they continue throwing the ball at the next letter and catch it. (Upgrade this activity by adding more letters or downgrade the activity by only placing two to three letters on the wall.)
- Child repeats a series of numbers, letters, or colors.
- Board games: Therapist plays board game with child. Child attempts to remember when their turn is, without verbal prompting from therapist.
- Child engages in different arts and crafts projects.
- Child sings parts of a song while performing an activity.
- Child sings a complete song for therapist.

- Freeze dancing: Child dances to music. When music stops, child freezes in place.
- Red Light, Green Light, 1, 2, 3: Therapist stands next to the wall with back facing the child. Therapist says "red light, green light, 1, 2, 3" and then turns to face the child. Child runs to touch therapist but stops once therapist turns around. If therapist catches child running, child must return to the wall and start again.
- Child jumps into ball pit. Therapist instructs the child to throw balls into a basket in specific order, differentiating the balls by color. For example, therapist instructs child to throw "red, blue, red, yellow" in that specific order.
- Bingo: Child plays Bingo in group or with therapist. (This game can be played with Bingo cards with numbers, shapes, or pictures in order to upgrade or downgrade level of difficulty).
- Card games: Therapist and child play card games together. Examples include gin, go fish, and war.
- Memory: Child and therapist play Memory game together.
- I Spy: Therapist plays I Spy with child in a small room (this will force the child to pay attention and look for details around the room.)
- Arrow Game: Therapist hides something in the room or inside the building. Therapist tapes arrows (created out of masking tape) on the floor leading to the hidden toy. Child follows arrows and peels each arrow off of the floor as they pass it.

Commercially Available Products

- Clue Junior
- Cranium Hullabaloo
- Hyper Dash
- Simon
- Stare!

Executive Functioning and Organizational Skills

Executive functioning refers to a neurocognitive process that includes planning, organizing, and decision making (Welsh & Pennington, 1988). In children, difficulties with organizational skills are most commonly seen in the school-based setting (Langberg et al., 2008). Some problems that will manifest themselves due to poor organization skills include forgetting homework assignments, losing school work, difficulty planning for long-term projects, difficulty studying for exams, and trouble keeping class materials organized (DuPaul & Stoner, 2014). Various interventions aimed at improving organizational skills have shown significant improvements in the areas of homework, time management, and planning for events in the future. Activities geared at improving organizational strategies are important to employ by themselves or coupled along with other evidence-based interventions (Langberg et al., 2008).

This chapter provides various activities that may be upgraded or downgraded based on the child's functional level and abilities. Demands placed on the child should be just slightly above the child's current ability, which research shows to be the optimal level for a child to learn. This level is called "the zone of proximal development," a concept developed by Russian psychologist Lev Vygotsky. This type of learning style enables a child to learn with assistance from someone who is more skilled and ultimately leads the child to achieve independence in the skill (Vygotsky, 1986).

ORGANIZATIONAL SKILLS ACTIVITIES

Following Set Directions

- Single-step direction following: Therapist creates a score sheet for child and gives them a sticker upon completing each direction correctly. (See Appendix A, p. 245, for sample sticker score card.) Single-step directions can focus on commands with prepositional use. Examples include "Place the penny IN the box," "Stand ON TOP OF the paper," "Walk AROUND the chair," and "Climb THROUGH the tunnel."

- Multiple-step direction-following: Child follows a three-step direction. For example, "Run to the door, skip to the basketball hoop, and shoot three baskets." Therapist grades direction's level of difficulty based on child's ability.

- Child completes color-by-number/color-by-letter handouts. (See Appendix A, pp. 246-251, for sample handouts.)

- Child copies block or building designs.

Danto, A. H., & Pruzansky, M. *1001 Pediatric Treatment Activities: Creative Ideas for Therapy Sessions, Third Edition* (pp. 143-144).
© 2023 SLACK Incorporated.

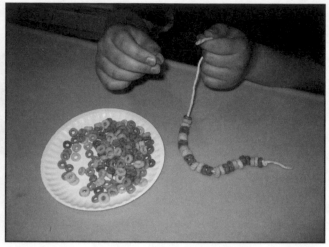

Figure 22-2.

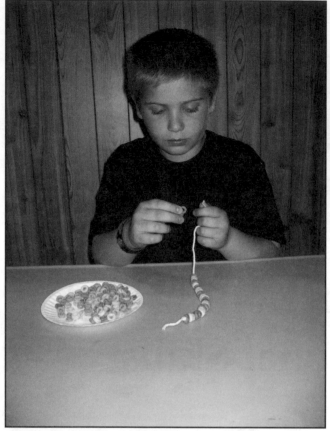

Figure 22-1.

- Child follows patterns with beads, pegs, or Froot Loops (Figures 22-1 and 22-2).

- Getting dressed: Therapist instructs the child to put on several articles of clothing in a specific order. For example, first socks, then shoes, then hat, then jacket, etc.

- Setting the table: Child follows either verbal or visual directions/instructions to set a table for mealtime.

- Following a recipe
  - Child completes a simple cooking project from a ready-to-bake mix.
  - Child follows a more difficult recipe from a cookbook, with assistance and supervision from the therapist as needed.

Strategizing

- Sudoku: This game requires strategy and concentration. Visit www.websudoku.com to print out very simple forms of the Sudoku puzzles.

- Scavenger hunt: Therapist creates a list of items child must find in the room. Child checks off each item once it is found. (See Appendix A, p. 252, for sample scavenger hunt.)

- Multiple-step obstacle course: Child completes a series of tasks in an obstacle course. Some examples include climbing through the tunnel, over the barrel, under the bean bag and jumping into the hoop, walking around the cones, hopping over the blocks, etc.

- Letter find obstacle course: Therapist tells child a letter. Child completes an obstacle course and at the end of the course finds the letter hidden among other letters hanging on the wall.

Commercially Available Products

- Battleship
- Connect Four
- Memory
- Othello
- Scrabble

VII

Social Skills

The complex social skills needed for a well-adjusted interaction with other children are among the most important skills a child must acquire. Deficits in social skills play a significant role in the development of many emotional and behavioral disorders of childhood and adolescence (Combs & Slaby, 1977). Additionally, children with poor social skills are more likely to develop adjustment problems as adults (Cowen et al., 1973). A child with poor social skills may find it challenging to participate in classroom activities, play a game with peers, or maintain eye contact when speaking with a friend (Williamson & Dorman, 2002).

Social skills training is directed at helping a child increase the ability to perform crucial social behaviors that are important in achieving success in social situations (Combs & Slaby, 1977). Social skill training will typically focus on teaching a child to engage in various interactions, interpersonal games, and social activities (Michelson et al., 2013).

This section will provide activities that promote social interactions and provide different games, group projects, group activities, and seasonal-based games and projects, all geared at improving social skills.

It is important to note that many of the activities provided work on multiple components of social competence, and it is at the discretion of the treating therapist to determine the primary area to work on with the child.

23

Increasing Social Interaction and Relatedness

In the school-based setting, a child will be faced with infinite social interactions including those at play time, recess, and collaborative academic work in the classroom (Schmidt et al., 2019). Appropriate social interactions enable a child to make friends and create relationships with peers. Social interactions also help teach children how to behave in a socially appropriate manner.

There are different components to appropriate social interactions and being related. Maintaining eye contact is one important part of being able to interact and relate with one's peers. Maintaining eye contact is often difficult, especially for children with an autism spectrum disorder (Carbone et al., 2013).

In addition to maintaining eye contact, there are also many other components of social competence that can be addressed while performing activities from this chapter. Some of these include reading facial expressions, understanding nonverbal social cues, maintaining appropriate personal space, modulating voice volume, having the ability to take turns, negotiating, and solving problems (Williamson & Dorman, 2002).

Although there are an infinite number of games and activities that can be played to help work on increasing a child's social skills, this chapter provides a sample of these sorts of activities. Many will require pairing children up and call for interdependence on the child's partner for suc-

cess in an activity. These activities should first be attempted with the child interacting with an adult. As the child comes closer to mastering an activity, they should then attempt the activity with another child.

INCREASING SOCIAL INTERACTION AND RELATEDNESS WITH CHILD AND PEERS

Back-and-Forth Games

- Roly poly: Therapist and child roll ball back and forth between them while sitting on floor with legs spread apart (Figure 23-1).

- Wonder ball/pass-the-ball-around game: Therapist and child pass ball back and forth between them while singing the wonder ball song. The song is sung as follows: "The wonder ball goes around and around, to pass it quickly you are bound, if you're the one to hold

Danto, A. H., & Pruzansky, M. *1001 Pediatric Treatment Activities: Creative Ideas for Therapy Sessions, Third Edition* (pp. 147-149).
© 2023 SLACK Incorporated.

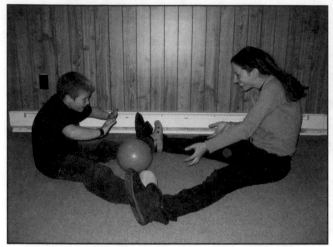

Figure 23-1.

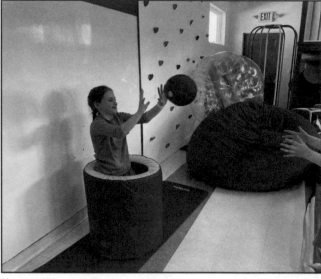

Figure 23-2.

it last, you will owe …" When ball stops, child and therapist perform an action together (e.g., touch their heads, clap hands).

- Ball games: Child sits in a chair or stands in a barrel (in order to stay stationary) and plays toss/catch games with therapist (Figure 23-2).

Interdependence Games

- Peek-a-Boo games: Child hides behind a pillow, under a small blanket, or in a tunnel and plays Peek-a-Boo with therapist.
- Scooter-board games
  - Child sits on a scooter holding onto a rope. Therapist pulls child on scooter by pulling the rope.
  - Two children sit on separate scooters. Therapist ties rope around the handle of two scooters. The children hold hands while being pulled.
  - Several children lie prone on scooter boards. Children make a train by holding onto the child's ankles in front of them. Therapist pulls rope tied onto the first scooter board.
- Chasing games: Child and therapist play tag and other chasing games together.

Group Games

In the following games, it is important to determine the appropriate level of involvement of the therapist, whether it be directly playing, supervising, or facilitating.

- Hide and Seek
- Simon Says
- Follow the Leader
- "Hokey Pokey"

- Freeze dance
- Musical Chairs
- Red Light, Green Light 1, 2, 3
- Card games: Gin, War, Go Fish
- Board games: Therapist chooses any board game that requires two or more players (eg, Checkers, Candy Land, Guess Who?).
- Four Corners: In this game, one person is designated the counter. All four corners of the room are numbered corners one through four. The counter stands in the middle of the room and counts to 10, while covering their eyes. While the counter is counting, the other children can run around the room and pick one of the corners to stand in. The counter then calls out a number between one and four, referring to one of the corners with their eyes still closed and then opens their eyes. All of the children who are standing in the corner called out are "out." Counter repeats counting until only one child is left. The last child left wins and gets to be the counter in the next round.

Sensory Activities With Movement, Touch, and Song

- "Ring Around the Rosie"
- "This Little Piggy …" (Figure 23-3)
- "Patty Cake," "Miss Mary Mack" (Figure 23-4)
- "Hot Potato" (Figures 23-5 and 23-6)
- "Itsy Bitsy Spider": Therapist sings song with child while trying to make eye contact.

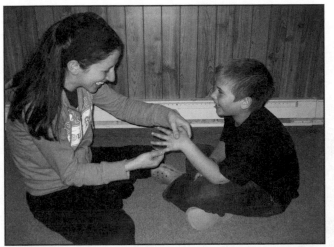

Figure 23-3.

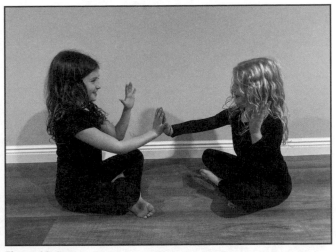

Figure 23-4.

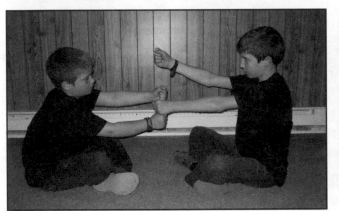

Figure 23-5.

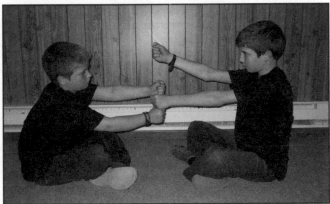

Figure 23-6.

- "If You're Happy and You Know It": Therapist sings this song with child. Child finishes each phrase and acts it out with therapist (e.g., "If you're happy and you know it … touch your nose").

- Therapist places child on swing and says "go" and "stop" when starting and stopping movement. Therapist attempts to have child say these words in order to direct therapist to move swing. Therapist can also try to have the child count "1, 2, 3" to direct therapist to swing the swing.

- Therapist places child on a therapy ball. Therapist bounces child on the ball while focusing on eye contact and increasing vocalizations and other sounds.

- Therapist provides linear vestibular movement on a platform swing while maintaining eye contact with child.

Making Eye Contact

- Therapist plays games with child in front of a mirror and makes eye contact through the mirror (e.g., therapist and child sing "Head, Shoulders, Knees, and Toes").

- Copy games: Child watches therapist and:
  - Imitates different facial expressions.
  - Imitates a beating pattern on a drum.
  - Imitates different funny body postures.

- Facial cues: Therapist makes different faces at child. Child tells therapist what emotion is being displayed (anger, sadness, happiness, surprise, etc.). Child then tries to imitate a specific emotion.

Commercially Available Products

- Guess Who?
- Twister

Group Activities

Group activities are a great way to help build social skills and friendship among children of all ages. Fun and exciting games and projects that can be played with two or more children are provided in this chapter. The treating therapist can choose to have the listed activities played between several children or between therapist and child. Some children with more severe social deficits will require an adult to prompt and guide them during many of these social activities.

In planning a group, it is important to understand the population one is working with and to know any specific child's needs in advance. This is to make sure that there will be enough adult supervision and assistance. A group's success often depends on adult supervision and assistance.

GROUP ACTIVITY THEMES

Funny Ball Games

- Over/under game: Children line up and pass a small ball between them. The first child passes it backward over their head, and the next child passes it backward between their legs. Once the last child gets the ball, all the children turn and face the opposite direction and play again (Figures 24-1 and 24-2).

- Funny passing game: Children sit in a circle and try to pass a small ball without using their hands. They can pass it by grabbing it with their elbows or feet, knocking it with their heads, or any other safe and creative way.

- Neck ball: Children pass a small ball from one child to the next without using their hands, passing it only with their necks (Figure 24-3).

Color-Themed Groups

- Color "Hokey Pokey": Therapist cuts out strips of tissue paper and gives children different colored strips. Children then sing the "Hokey Pokey" song: "Put your red hand in," etc. After this is done with tissue paper, it can also be done with small balls or different colored bean bags.

- Therapist covers a flashlight with different pieces of colored Cellophane wrap. Therapist turns out the lights and shines each color on the ceiling, then asks each child to find one item in the given color. Children bring their items into the middle of the circle.

Danto, A. H., & Pruzansky, M. *1001 Pediatric Treatment Activities: Creative Ideas for Therapy Sessions, Third Edition* (pp. 151-158).
© 2023 SLACK Incorporated.

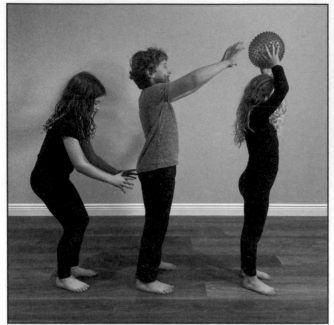

Figure 24-1.

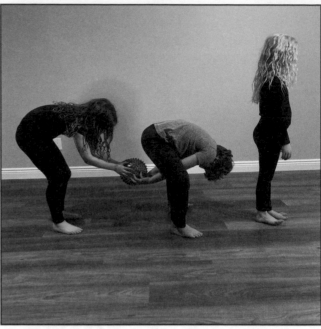

Figure 24-2.

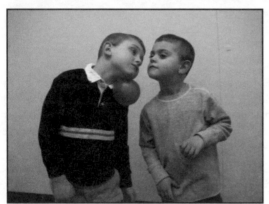

Figure 24-3.

- Color hunt: Children close their eyes and pick a piece of colored construction paper out of a bag filled with small pieces of construction paper in various colors. Each child tries to find something of that color in the room.

- "If You're Wearing …": Play a Simon Says style game (e.g., "If you're wearing red, stand up. If you're wearing blue, clap your hands.").

- Color-association game: Therapist places index cards with fruit, animals, clothing, etc., of various colors on a board in front of the children. Children take turns sorting these cards into the correct color categories.

- I Spy: Children play the I Spy game using colors as clues. For example, therapist says, "I spy something red that is on the top shelf of the bookcase." Children then try to guess that object.

- Building a colored tower: Children pick a color out of a hat and then add the corresponding colored block to a tower. Children see how tall they can make the tower before it falls.

- Child picks a color out of a hat and then hops/jumps/wheelbarrow-walks to something matching the same color across room.

Letter-Themed Groups

- Therapist places several index cards with letters on a wall, orienting the cards in different directions (some cards will be upright, upside down, sideways, diagonal, etc.). Therapist chooses a random word. Child throws a ball against the wall onto the first letter of the word and then catches it as it bounces back. Child continues to throw the ball against the wall onto the second and then remaining letters of the word and then catches it.

- Letter-themed obstacle course: Child picks a letter out of a hat and looks at it, but therapist holds onto it. Child then completes the obstacle course. At the end of the obstacle course, several letters should be hanging on a wall either in the same case or in a different case (upper or lower). Child identifies the chosen letter on the wall and then tapes it on top of the matching letter on the wall (Figure 24-4).

- Each child builds the letters of their name out of pegs. Therapist mixes all the assembled letters together and spreads them out on the floor. Each child individually walks to find the letters of their name and then spells it out on a table (Figures 24-5 and 24-6).

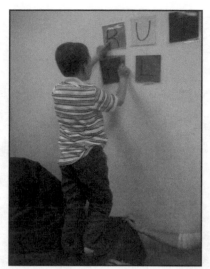

Figure 24-4.

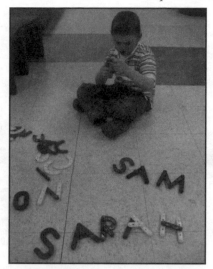

Figure 24-5.

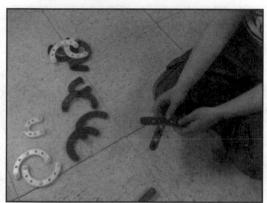

Figure 24-6.

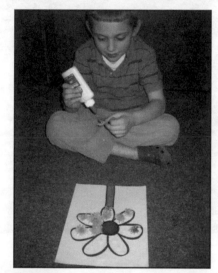

Figure 24-7.

Number-Themed Groups

- Children go outside and collect small leaves or flowers. They are given a page showing a picture of an empty tree or flower, onto which they then glue the leaves or flower petals. Children count up the number of leaves/petals on the tree or flower and write that number on the tree trunk/flower stem (Figures 24-7 and 24-8).

- Number chart: Children are given the number chart (see Appendix A, p. 253) and then asked to glue the corresponding number of sequins or foam pieces onto the row (Figures 24-9 and 24-10).

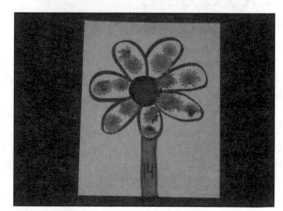

Figure 24-8.

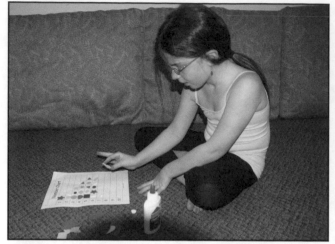

Figure 24-9.

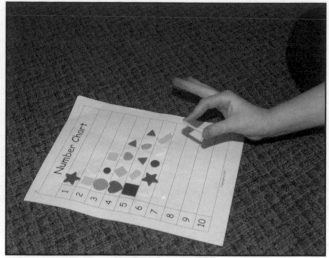

Figure 24-10.

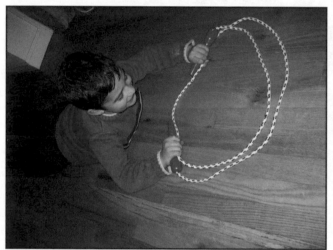

Figure 24-11.

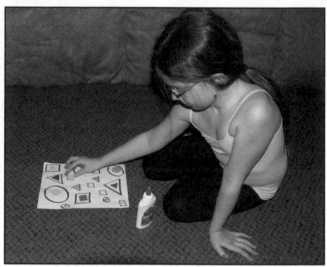

Figure 24-12.

Shapes Groups

- Therapist places different shapes all over the floor around the room. Therapist gives the children gross motor instructions regarding the shapes. For example, therapist may say, "Jump over the squares, hop over the triangles, march around the rectangles," etc.

- Therapist places items of various shapes into a bag (square book, triangle puzzle piece, ball, etc.). Children stick their hands into the bag and use stereognosis (i.e., the ability to identify objects based on touch without the assistance of vision) to determine what shape they are touching.

- Children make shapes out of a jump rope (Figure 24-11).

- Children try to make shapes with their fingers. They then lie on the floor and position their bodies to make specific shapes. With an instant print camera or digital camera, therapist takes a picture of the children once they are in the correct position.

- Shape instructions: Therapist provides each child with a shape handout (see shape instruction handout in Appendix A, p. 254). Children follow the key at the bottom of the page. Instructions include make dots in the circles, make vertical lines in the triangles, and make horizontal lines in the squares.

- Shape collage: Therapist makes large circles, squares, rectangles, and any other shape all over a piece of paper and then gives out craft foam pieces. Children glue the corresponding shapes into the large shapes on the paper (Figure 24-12). An alternative activity would be to have the children just draw smaller shapes into the large ones (Figure 24-13).

- Children create pictures solely out of cutout shapes (e.g., of a person, house, ice cream cone; Figure 24-14).

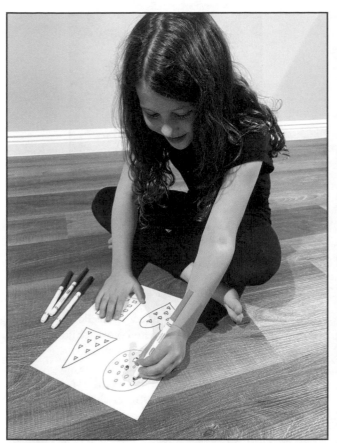

Figure 24-13.

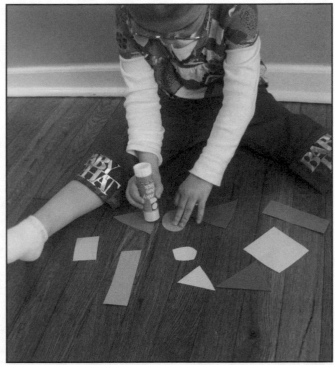

Figure 24-14.

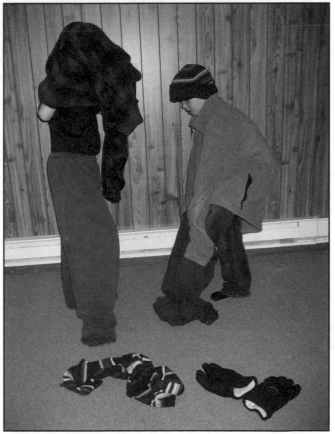

Figure 24-15.

Teamwork Games

- Relay races: Examples include three-legged race, potato sack race, placing a spoon in mouth with an egg or ping-pong ball on the spoon, transferring water from one bucket to another, frog jumping, backward walking, twirling, etc.

- Clothing race: Therapist places different articles of oversized clothing on one side of the room. Children must race to the other side of the room and get dressed in the large T-shirt, shorts, and socks as quickly as possible (Figures 24-15 and 24-16).

- Scavenger hunt: Children play the game together as a group in a circle. Child gets a turn to find one item on the list and bring it back into the circle. Alternatively, small groups can be formed and the children can play in teams against one another. (See Appendix A, p. 252, for a sample scavenger hunt.)

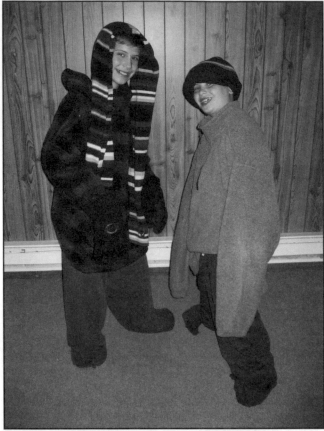

Figure 24-16.

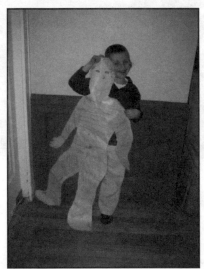

Figure 24-18.

Building Social Skills

- Get to know you game: Children are given an empty sticker chart (see Appendix A, p. 245, for the sticker chart). Each child picks a category card with a question on it at random out of a bag. Child then asks one friend

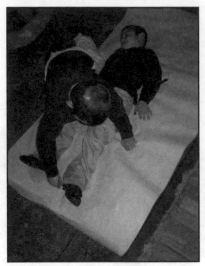

Figure 24-17.

in the circle to answer this question. For example, if the category picked is favorite colors, child must ask someone in the circle, "What is your favorite color?" and then be able to tell the group the answer. For each correct question and answer, both children are given a small sticker to place on the sticker chart.

- Mummy wrap: Children pair up in teams of two or more people. One child is designated to be the "mummy." The mummy must stand still while other children in group wrap toilet paper around them.

- Human puppet game: Therapist pairs up children. Therapist places large pieces of paper on floor. One child from each pair lies on paper. Other child traces out the body outline. Children then switch. After this is completed, children cut out their puppets (with therapist assistance if needed), draw or glue on body parts, and decorate them (Figures 24-17 and 24-18).

- Children make hand puppets out of brown paper bags. Children glue on googly eyes, color in the mouth, and put on feathers for hair. Children sing songs and talk to each other using their puppets (Figure 24-19).

- "Bridge-body-connect"
  - Several children perform a bridge with their backs (therapist assistance may be required). Remaining children crawl under all of the other children's bridges (Figure 24-20).
  - Therapist then pairs up the children in groups of two. Children lie on their backs on the floor with their feet touching their partner's feet. Both children raise their legs off of the floor and press their feet against the partner's feet (Figure 24-21). Remaining children crawl under the bridge.

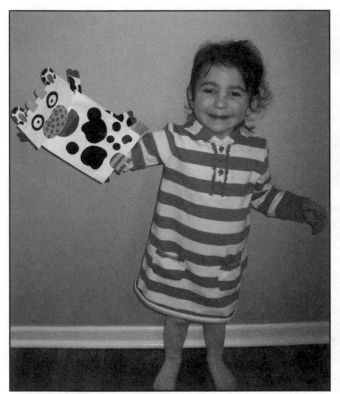

Figure 24-19.

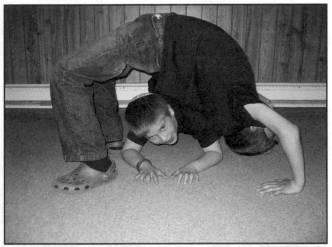

Figure 24-20.

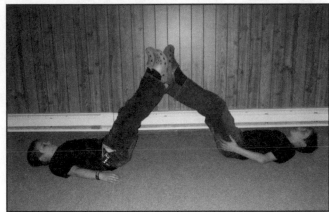

Figure 24-21.

○ Children then face each other and hold hands. Children raise their hands so other children can climb under. (Think of other fun and creative ways to connect the children's bodies and make more bridges.)

- Telephone: Children sit in a circle. One child or therapist whispers a word or sentence into the next child's ear. That child whispers what they heard to the next child. Finally, the last child says what they heard out loud, and the original person says whether or not that was correct.

- Cookie making: Therapist takes cookies and has children spread icing on them with their fingers. Children then decorate their cookies with sprinkles, small pretzel pieces, raisins, etc. Each child makes two cookies, one for themselves and one for a friend.

- "Ring Around the Rosie"

- Rolling game: Children all lie on their backs on a mat next to each other. They sing the song, "There were [insert number] children in a bed and the little one said roll over." Children continuously roll without touching the next child while singing the song; they freeze once they reach the edge of the mat. Children then continue rolling the other way.

Groups to Work on Attention and Organization

- Random association groups: Children match pictures or words to something associated with them (e.g., summer/hot, dog/bone, bed/pillow, raindrop/umbrella).

- Association groups based on seasons and holidays. Therapist creates cards with association pictures/words. Children play matching and sorting games with cards.

- Memory: Children play Memory games in a group.

- Bingo: Children play Bingo together. Children can use numbers, shapes, or pictures in Bingo. Therapist can create Bingo sheets with a few items on the page or many in order to upgrade or downgrade the level of difficulty.

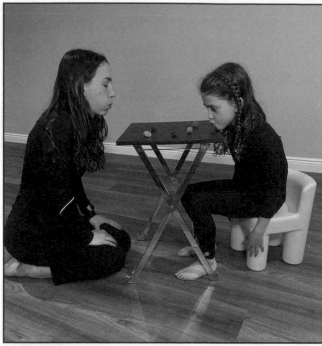

Figure 24-22.

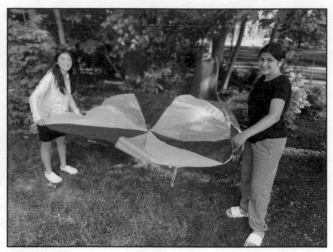

Figure 24-23.

Sensory Groups

- Sensory baseball: Child comes up to bat either on a tee or be thrown a slow pitch. Child hits the ball and runs around the bases. Each base should be a sensory activity. For example, first base could be a trampoline that you have to jump on 10 times. Second base could be a large bean bag that the child crashes into. Third base could be a wedge that child must crawl up and jump off, etc.

- Oral motor group

  ○ Therapist places a pom-pom on the table. Children blow the pom-pom back and forth between them without letting the pom-pom fall off the table (Figure 24-22).

  ○ Children can also each be given whistles and take turns blowing them. After this, the therapist can hold an empty paper towel roll and sing a song through it (using it as a microphone). Therapist should only start the song, and the children should pass around the "microphone" and take turns saying the specific verse in the song.

- Pin the tail on the donkey: Children can play this game with eyes open, closed, spinning, and no spinning.

- Parachute games: Children walk holding onto parachute handles, run underneath parachute when it is raised, sit on the middle of parachute, and be pulled by therapists (Figure 24-23).

- Parachute popcorn game: Children crumple large strips of tissue paper and throw them into the middle of the parachute. Once all the colors are in the middle, children swing the parachute up and down and watch the "popcorn." They try to keep the popcorn from falling off the sides for as long as possible (Figure 24-24).

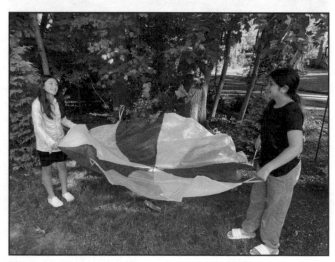

Figure 24-24.

25

Seasonally Themed Projects and Activities

The different seasons offer times for learning and fun. This chapter provides various activities and projects that can be completed during the different seasons. When selecting a project or activity, it is important to keep in mind the child's abilities and the specific skills that need to be strengthened.

Because many teachers and therapists work with a variety of children from different backgrounds, it is important to keep in mind cultural and religious sensitivities before selecting a project or activity.

FALL ACTIVITIES

- Games
  - Pin the stem on the pumpkin: Draw a very large pumpkin without a stem on a piece of oak tag or paper. Cut a stem out of green construction paper. Place adhesive on the back of the stem. Blindfold the children and have them take turns trying to place the stem on the correct spot on the pumpkin (same rules as with pin the tail on the donkey).

Therapist must use sound judgment in selecting a blindfold activity with a specific child and must carefully supervise any activity involving blindfolding.

- Apple bowling: Place pictures of apples on bowling pins. Have the children roll a ball and try to knock over the pins (if bowling pins are not available, small cones can be used).

- Fall Bingo: Create a fall Bingo sheet. Categories can include apples, pumpkins, acorns, leaves, pine cones, and trees with fall-colored leaves. Have children play Bingo in a group.

- Fall Memory: Create small cards with fall-themed pictures. Make two of each. Mix the cards together and place them facedown on the table. Then have the children play fall Memory. (Sample categories are included in the fall Bingo activity.)

- Turkey hunt: Make photocopies of a picture of a turkey. Hide the turkeys around the room and ask the children to find the hidden turkeys. After one round, split the children into two groups. Have one group of children hide the turkeys and then allow the other group to search for them (then switch hider and finder groups.)

Danto, A. H., & Pruzansky, M. *1001 Pediatric Treatment Activities: Creative Ideas for Therapy Sessions, Third Edition* (pp. 159-162). © 2023 SLACK Incorporated.

○ Fall gross motor activity: Create two sets of matching fall cards (sample categories provided in the fall Bingo activity). Spread the two piles on opposite sides of the room. Instruct a child to pick a specific card from the first pile and then have the child go the other pile while following a gross motor instruction (e.g., hop, jump, skip, gallop, wheelbarrow-walk, crab-walk, scooter, backward walk, frog-jump).

○ Leaves hunt: Go outside and search for different types of leaves.

○ Visit the website http://www.dltk-holidays.com. From it you can automatically create Bingo sheets, Memory cards, and other holiday-themed games.

- Projects

  ○ Cut out and color pumpkin shapes, then hide them around the room and have a pumpkin hunt where the children must find their friends' hidden pumpkins.

  ○ Tissue paper corn project: Create a corn template and ask children to cut it out. Have long pieces of green tissue paper and small pieces of yellow tissue paper. Ask children to glue on the long green pieces for the husk, then take one yellow piece of tissue paper in each hand and crumple them up. Glue the yellow tissue paper pieces in the middle for the kernels. Continue crumpling and gluing until the entire template is covered with tissue paper.

  ○ Scarecrow project: Give each child five pieces of a scarecrow that have to be put together in the correct order. Each child should be given a cutout pumpkin head, straw body, pants, shoes, and straw hat (the body parts can also be photocopied and cut out by the children themselves).

  ○ Acorn maracas: Ask children to collect acorns from outside. Color and decorate two paper plates. Staple the plates together with the tops of the plates facing each other. Do not staple all the way around so that there is some space left with a hole to put in the acorns. Give each child acorns and have them put the acorns inside the holes. Then staple the plates all the way so there is no space for the acorns to fall out. The children can play with and shake their maracas to the beat of a tune.

  ○ Pumpkin decorating: Provide small pumpkins and allow the children to decorate them with markers, paint, sequins, feathers, etc.

  ○ Hand turkeys: Trace each child's hand on brown construction paper to make a turkey. Glue feathers onto the fingertips and a googly eye onto the thumb.

○ Fruit turkeys: Place an orange or an apple sideways on the table. Place four toothpicks on the top of the fruit and one toothpick into the side of the fruit. (The toothpicks will serve as feathers and the head.) Stick four raisins into each toothpick on the turkey's back and one grape on the turkey's head. Then place one mini marshmallow on the top of each of the four toothpicks on the turkey's back.

○ Thankful turkey project: Ask the children to glue colorful tissue paper onto the back of a paper plate, which will serve as the turkey's back. Give each child four pieces of construction paper that have been cut into the shapes of turkey feathers. Ask the children to write one thing that they are thankful for on each feather. Then glue the feathers onto the plate. Place googly eyes and draw on a nose.

○ Book of thanks: Ask the children to create a book of thanks by writing a different word or sentence on each page about something they are thankful for. Then let the children illustrate their book of thanks. To bind the pages of the book together, punch holes on the edges of the paper and then tie string or yarn through them (the book can also be stapled together).

○ Hand trees: Therapist paints child's arm and hand with brown and green paint, respectively. Child presses down on paper to form the trunk and leaves of the tree. Child dips fingertips into paint of the different fall colors. Child then makes dots on paper to finger-paint leaves all over the tree.

○ Leaf shading: Collect leaves from the ground outdoors. Place the leaves under a piece of white paper. With a crayon, color lightly on the paper over the leaf. The shape of a leaf will then appear on the paper.

WINTER ACTIVITIES

- Games

  ○ Visit the website http://www.dltk-holidays.com. There you can automatically create Bingo sheets, Memory cards, and other holiday-themed games.

  ○ Bundle up the bear: To work on dressing skills, have a child dress a stuffed animal with winter clothes, using infant's clothing. It can be made into a game of "we pass the bear around" and, each time the bear stops, another article of clothing is added.

  ○ Indoor sledding: Have child sit on a scooter-board while holding onto a jump rope with two hands; an adult or another child can pull the rope to propel the child around the room.

- ○ Winter Bingo: Create a winter Bingo sheet. Sample categories can include snowman, sled, jacket, ice-skating, skiing etc. Then have children play Bingo in a group.

- ○ Winter Memory: Create small cards with winter-themed pictures. Make two of each. Mix the cards up and place them facedown on the table. Then have the children play winter Memory. (Sample categories are included in the winter Bingo activity.)

- Projects

  - ○ Snowman: Make a snowman using three small white paper plates. Cut out an orange triangle for the mouth, glue on buttons for the eyes, and use crumpled tissue paper balls to form the mouth. Staple on brown pipe cleaners for the arms.

  - ○ Snowflake projects: Fold a white paper in half several times, then snip different shapes with scissors. Unfold the paper to see the snowflake. It can be decorated with glitter for a sparkle effect.

  - ○ Handprint evergreen tree with snow: Therapist paints green finger paint on child's hands. Child makes multiple upside-down handprints on a large paper in the shape of an evergreen tree (triangle). If necessary, a triangular border can be drawn on the paper for the child prior to the painting. Therapist then makes a mixture of half glue/half shaving cream. Child paints mixture on tree to get a puffy "snow" effect when dry.

  - ○ Create calendars: Have children draw pictures associated with each month of the year. Print out calendar pages for the 12 months of the year. Place a picture above each month and staple the calendar together.

SPRING ACTIVITIES

- Games

  - ○ Children go into potato sacks and pop up and down out of the potato sacks, pretending to be flowers blooming. They then have a potato sack race.

  - ○ Flowers Memory game: Create flower Memory cards by coloring matches of different sorts of flowers on the cards. Then have the children play a game of Memory.

  - ○ Visit the website http://www.dltk-holidays.com. There you can automatically create Bingo sheets, Memory cards, and other holiday-themed games.

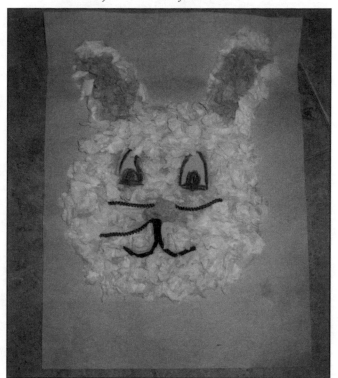

Figure 25-1.

- Projects

  - ○ Pop-up ground hog on a Popsicle stick: Print out picture of groundhogs. Have the children color them and glue them to Popsicle sticks to make puppets. For each puppet, cut out two squares of brown paper and staple them together on opposite sides (leaving the top and bottom open). Put the puppet into the "pocket underground" and then make it pop up.

  - ○ Make bunnies: Create a blank template of a rabbit on a piece of construction paper. Ask the children to place small pieces of Styrofoam or crumpled white and pink tissue paper on the bunny. Then make the mouth and whiskers with black pipe cleaners (Figure 25-1).

  - ○ Bunny hats: Cut out hats with bunny ears and place on the children's heads. Then tell the children to hop around the room like bunnies.

  - ○ Tissue paper flowers: Cut four to six pieces of tissue paper into 8- by 10-inch pieces. Place the pieces on top of each other and fold them like an accordion. Tie the center of the folded tissue paper with a green pipe cleaner. Then slowly unravel each layer one at a time, creating the flower's petals.

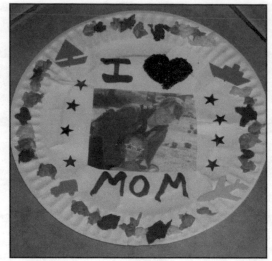

Figure 25-2.

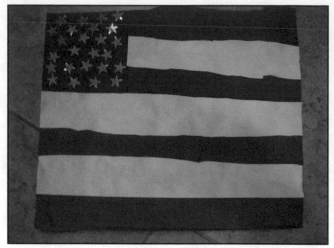

Figure 25-3.

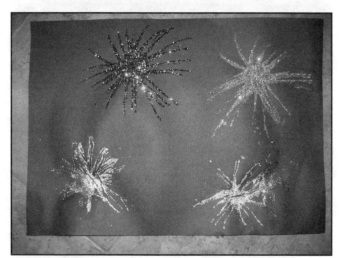

Figure 25-4.

○ Flower vases: Children paint and decorate empty water bottles or seltzer bottles with sequins. They can also wrap yarn or string of various colors around bottles.

○ Paper plate picture frames: Ask the children to bring in pictures of themselves with their mothers. Each child then cuts a hole in the center of his or her plate slightly smaller than the picture. It may be helpful to trace a line for the children and start the first cut so that the child does not rip the paper. Ask the children to decorate the plates with glitter, stickers, sequins, or other craft materials. Last, have an adult staple the pictures onto the plates from behind (Figure 25-2).

SUMMER ACTIVITIES

- Games
  ○ Summer Bingo: Create a summer Bingo sheet. Sample categories can include American flags, barbecues, hot dogs, hamburgers, ketchup, grills, fireworks, beach, sun, swimming, suntan lotion, ice cream, etc. Then have children play Bingo in a group.
  ○ Summer Memory: Create small cards with summer-themed pictures. Make two of each. Mix the cards together and place them facedown on the table. Then, have the children play summer Memory. (Sample categories are included in the summer Bingo activity.)

- Projects
  ○ American flags: Draw an American flag template on white paper. Cut out red strips and glue them to every other stripe. Cut out a blue square for the corner and use either small star stickers or silver glitter for the stars (Figure 25-3).
  ○ Watercolor fireworks: Provide each child with different colored paint in cups. Have the children squeeze the paint from the cup into a medicine dispenser and then create droplets on a white piece of paper. Next, have the children blow through a straw onto the paint droplets to create fireworks.
  ○ Glitter fireworks: Have children glue shooting lines onto a black piece of construction paper and then sprinkle glitter onto the lines (Figure 25-4).
  ○ American flag safety pin: Place small red, white, and blue beads onto the safety pin in the pattern of the American flag.

VIII

Improving Gait Patterns

Most children begin walking around 1 year of age with a wide base of support, a "foot-flat to foot-flat" pattern, and straight knees. By approximately the age of 3.5 years, children develop more mature gait patterns (Jacobs, 2010). However, some children will develop difficulties establishing mature gait because of various physical problems. Some problems include flat feet, increased internal rotation of the hips, increased external rotation of the hips, and/or toe-walking. A trained therapist can perform an assessment to determine if these issues are normal variants of development or require further evaluation and treatment (Jacobs, 2010).

In the upcoming chapters of this section, activities will be provided that address flat feet, increased internal rotation of the hips, increased external rotation of the hips, and/or toe-walking.

Increasing the Arches of the Foot

Flat feet can result from combined foot and ankle deformities. In addition to heel misalignment, a decreased arch is present as well (Kwon & Myerson, 2010). Approximately 4% of children at the age of 10 years have flat feet (Bertani et al., 1999), which can sometimes be due to decreased muscle strength (Andreasen et al., 2013). However, a flat foot can have other causes as well. Flat feet in children are often associated with pain, poor motor skills, altered gait patterns, and discomfort (Müller et al., 2012). Therefore, children with flat feet will have difficulty engaging in various sports and other age-appropriate activities because of this condition.

In this chapter, various activities are provided—including stretching, strengthening, and sensory activities—to help increase the arches of the foot.

INCREASING ARCHES OF THE FOOT

Activities Involving Balance

- Child stands barefoot on air disc and:
  ○ Maintains stationary balance.
  ○ Catches ball.
  ○ Moves slightly from side to side.
  ○ Stands in place and moves feet from pronated to supinated position.
- Child stands on one foot while resting other foot on the ball positioned on the floor. Child tries to maintain balance while singing the ABCs. (Upon completion, the position should be reversed, with opposite foot on ball.)

Danto, A. H., & Pruzansky, M. *1001 Pediatric Treatment Activities: Creative Ideas for Therapy Sessions, Third Edition* (pp. 165-168).
© 2023 SLACK Incorporated.

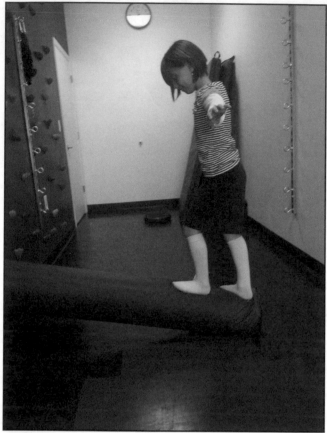

Figure 26-1.

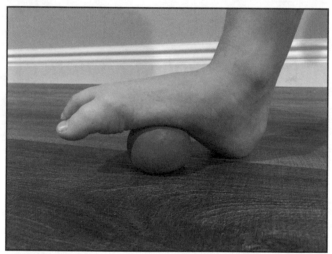

Figure 26-3.

- Bolster activities
  - Child stands with one foot on bolster and one foot on floor and maintains balance.
  - Child stands with one foot on bolster and one foot on floor and plays catch with therapist.

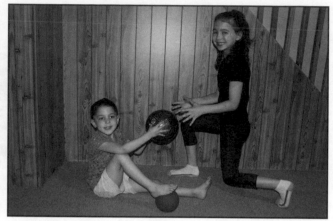

Figure 26-2.

- Child stands with one foot on bolster and one foot on floor. Child reaches to pick up nearby objects off floor on outside of the foot child is balancing on.
- Therapist places bolster on incline against wall. Child walks up bolster slowly (Figure 26-1).

Curling the Feet and Toes Around Objects

- Child picks up small Koosh balls around feet using only toes to pick them up. Child places them into nearby container with toes.
- Child stands on foam surface or soft pillows focusing on curving foot over surface.
- Child sits on floor with one foot placed on ball on floor and plays game with therapist or another child (Figure 26-2).
- Barefoot child rolls arches of foot over a tennis ball (Figure 26-3).

Foot Exercises and Stretches

- Theraband activities
  - Child sits in long sitting position. Therapist wraps Theraband around feet of child, mostly under the toes.
  - Child pushes Theraband forward with toes and holds for 5 seconds. Repeat 10 times (Figure 26-4).
- Therapist places a sticker on wall at height of child's nose. Child stands at arm's length from a wall with palms flat against the wall. Child slowly bends elbows to lean toward the wall trying to touch nose to sticker while keeping hips, knees, and back straight and heels flat on floor (Figure 26-5).

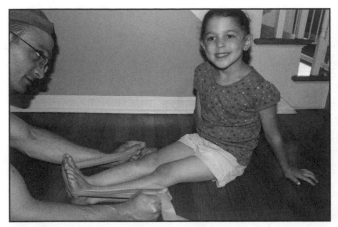

Figure 26-4.

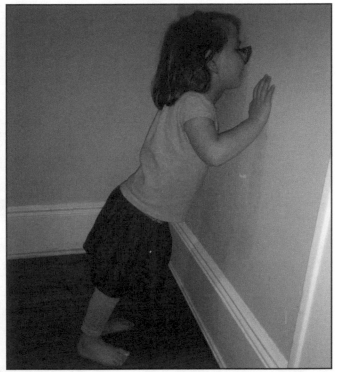

Figure 26-5.

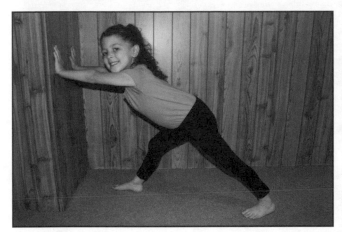

Figure 26-6.

- Barefoot movement: Child walks or runs barefoot across room several times.
- Achilles tendon stretching exercises
  - Child pushes against wall with one leg in front of other and back leg straight (Figure 26-6).
  - Child places one foot on curb and one foot on ground and bends down to touch curb (Figure 26-7).
- Foot/toe curling exercises
  - Child sits in long sitting position. They then plantar flex ankle and hold position for 5 seconds. Child then curls toes and holds position for 5 seconds. Repeat 10 times.
  - Child sits in long sitting position. They then curl just toes for 5 seconds and hold position. Repeat 10 times.
  - Child stands barefoot on a flat surface and tries to touch each toe to the floor one at a time. Therapist says "This Little Piggy" rhyme for each corresponding toe that child presses down.

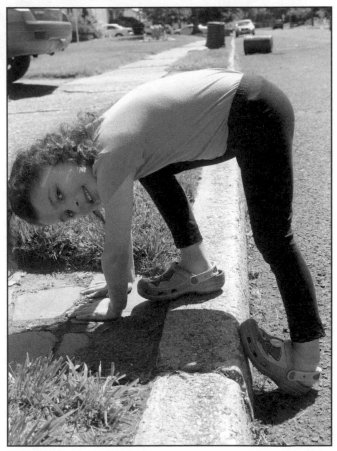

Figure 26-7.

Textured Surfaces Under the Foot

- Sandbox activities
  - Child walks back and forth across sandbox.
  - Child walks on sand and presses feet firmly into the sand, focusing on arch of foot.
  - Child stands on sand and curls foot on sand, making marks in sand.
  - Child stands in place and then rocks onto toes, freezes in place, and then rocks onto heels and freezes in place. Repeat 10 times.
  - Child stands in place and then rocks onto the side of the foot and holds position. They then rest feet flat on floor and repeat.
  - Child stands in sand and plays catch with therapist. Therapist tries to throw ball slightly off center to child so that child can focus on balance while standing in sand.
- Rice box activities
  - Child stands barefoot in rice box and curls foot in rice.
  - Child sits by edge of rice box and picks up small items with toes inside rice box.

Decreasing External Rotation of the Hips

Young children learning to walk will demonstrate gradual and progressively improved gait patterns between the ages of 1 and 3 years. By age 3 years, the amount of external rotation present in gait will be significantly decreased (Effgen, 2005). However, some children will continue to present with externally rotated hips, walking with a toe-out gait. External rotation of the hips can be caused by weak muscles or other musculoskeletal problems (Cibulka et al., 2010). Before treating children with externally rotated hips (or a toe-out gait), it is important to determine whether the problem stems from the hips or whether it is secondary to tibial torsion or torsion of the foot. It is also important to determine whether the amount of external rotation is part of normal development or an issue to be concerned about.

Externally rotated hips may affect balance and can make it difficult for a child to run, play, and engage in many age-appropriate activities. Asymmetry in hip rotation (where external rotation is greater than internal rotation or vice versa) is also associated with numerous musculoskeletal problems (Cibulka et al., 2010). Children who remain in hip external rotation for prolonged lengths of time will develop overstretched internal hip rotators and shortened or contracted external rotators.

This chapter provides various strengthening and stretching exercises. One of its main focuses is to enable the child to perform activities with tibial advancement over a fixed foot facing forward. The treating therapist should ensure proper musculoskeletal alignment in performing all of these activities in order to achieve the desired effect.

DECREASING EXTERNAL ROTATION OF THE HIPS

To promote tibial advancement over a fixed foot, have child do activities to target tibial progression over the foot.

Dynamic Strengthening Activities

- Side-walking (developmental age of 12 to 15 months): Therapist brings child near a couch or another long surface. Therapist places various toys along couch and has child side step to gather toys and place them into container. Therapist keeps child's hips and feet aligned throughout if needed (Figures 27-1 and 27-2).

Danto, A. H., & Pruzansky, M. *1001 Pediatric Treatment Activities:
Creative Ideas for Therapy Sessions, Third Edition* (pp. 169-174).
© 2023 SLACK Incorporated.

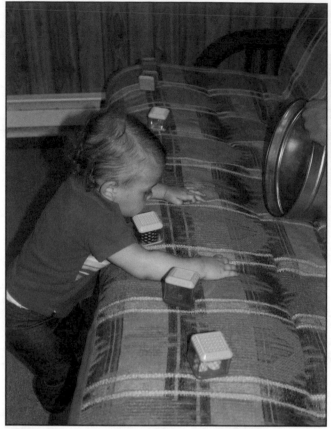

Figure 27-1.

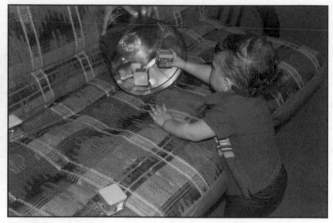

Figure 27-2.

- Squatting activity (developmental age of 12 to 15 months): Therapist has child stand next to pile of toys on floor. Child squats to pick up one toy at a time and place it into a container on a higher surface (Figure 27-3).
- Stair activities (Therapist must ensure proper alignment of hips during activity.)
  - Child steps up single step forward.
  - Child steps up single step to the side.
  - Child steps down single step backward.
- Tandem-walking activities
  - Child walks on a taped line across the floor.
  - Child walks across balance beam.
  - Child walks along curb outside.
- Seated scooter activities
  - Child sits on rolling scooter and propels scooter forward using feet only.
  - Child sits on rolling scooter and propels scooter with feet while picking up scattered objects around room (Figure 27-4).
- Jumping activities (Therapist helps child focus on foot placement during jumping activities; verbal and gentle physical cues may be needed.)
  - Child jumps up and down off the ground.
  - Child jumps over small object placed on the floor.
  - Child jumps with ball squeezed between knees.
- Wall slide: Child sits with hips at 90 degrees and back against wall. Child slides up and down wall (Figures 27-5 and 27-6).

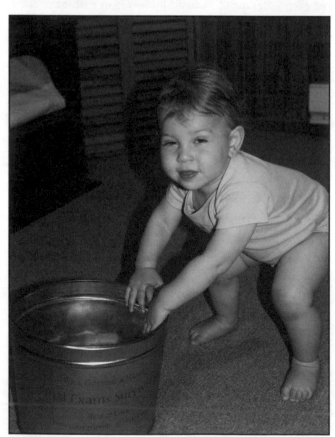

Figure 27-3.

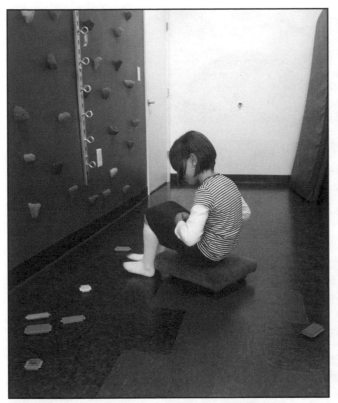

Figure 27-4.

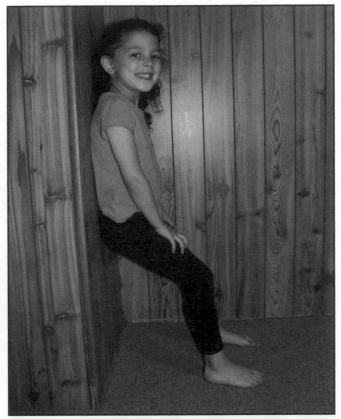

Figure 27-5.

- Knee kicking
  - Child drops medium-sized ball onto their knee and kicks it forward (Figure 27-7).
  - Child drops therapy ball onto their knee and kicks it forward (Figure 27-8).
  - Therapist slowly drops medium-sized ball over child's lower extremity. Child bounces ball off knee (Figure 27-9).
- Heel-walking: Child walks across room on heels.

Stationary Strengthening Activities

- Single-limb stance activities
  - Child balances on one foot.
  - Child stands with one foot on medium-sized ball and other foot aligned flat on floor.
- Dynadisc activities
  - Child stands on Dynadisc and maintains balance for X number of seconds (amount of time should be determined by treating therapist; Figure 27-10).
  - Child catches ball on Dynadisc.

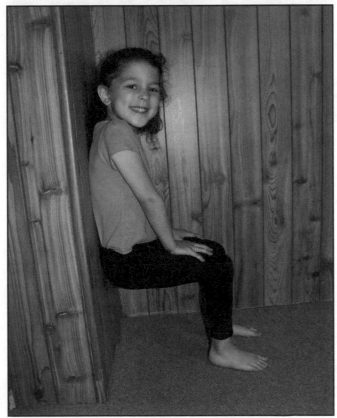

Figure 27-6.

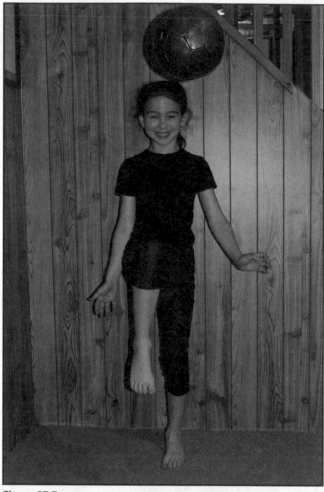

Figure 27-7.

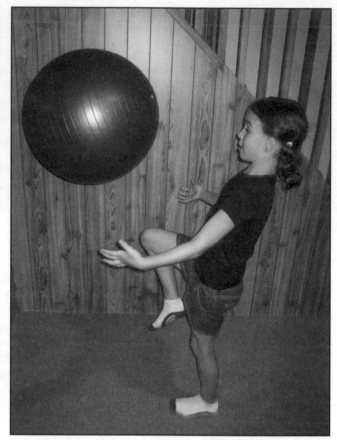

Figure 27-8.

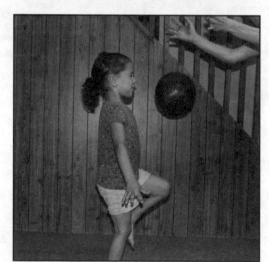

Figure 27-9.

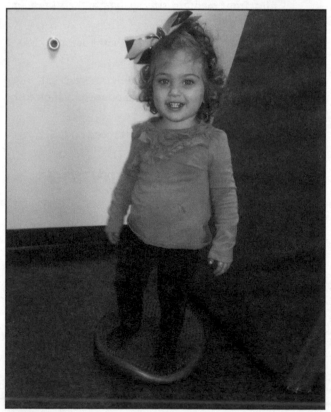

Figure 27-10.

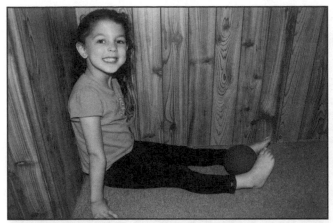

Figure 27-11.

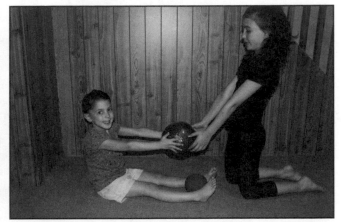

Figure 27-12.

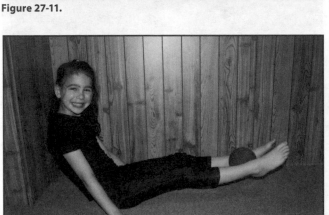

Figure 27-13.

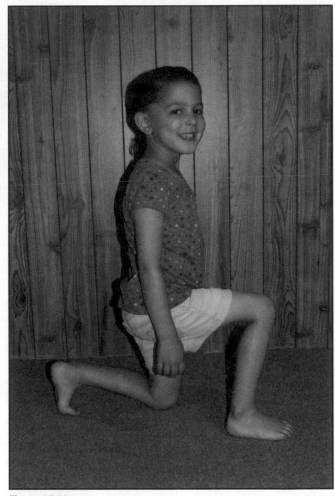

Figure 27-14.

- Activities in long sit with small or medium sized ball placed between the ankles.

Do not use a large ball or you may increase external rotation.

- Child squeezes and releases ball 10 times (Figure 27-11).
- Child squeezes ball and plays catch with therapist or another child with a different ball (Figure 27-12).
- Child places squeaky ball between ankles and squeezes toy to make it squeak and make noise.
- Child squeezes ball between ankles with straight legs slightly raised in air (Figure 27-13).

- Half-kneel activities
- Child maintains half-kneel position on the floor (Figure 27-14).
- Child pushes/pulls Theraband or rope in this position (Figure 27-15).
- Child moves from half-kneel position to stand (Figure 27-16).

- Child moves from half-kneel to tall-kneel position (Figure 27-17).
- Child reaches for objects all around and crossing midline (Figure 27-18).

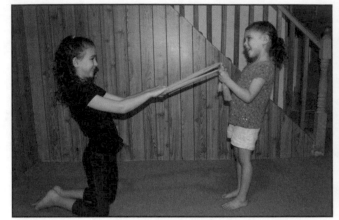

Figure 27-15.

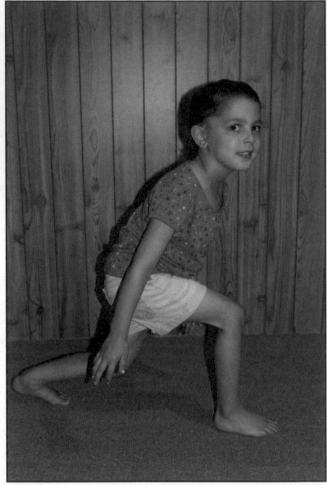

Figure 27-16.

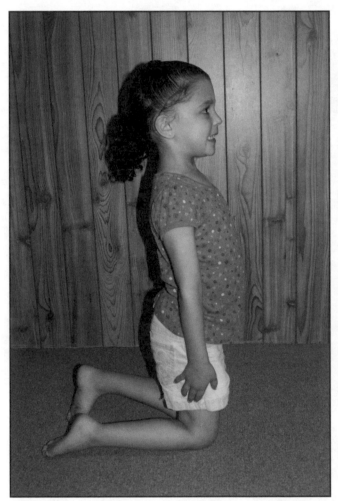

Figure 27-17.

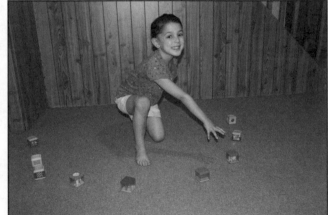

Figure 27-18.

Decreasing Internal Rotation of the Hips

28

Increased internal rotation of the hips is commonly found in children with spastic cerebral palsy (Wren et al., 2005). However, increased internal rotation can also be the result of weak external rotators (Cibulka et al., 2010) or other orthopedic conditions. Children who remain in internal rotation for prolonged lengths of time will develop overstretched external rotators and shortened or contracted internal rotators. These children will thus have difficulty walking, running, engaging in sports, and other gross motor activities. As stated in the introduction to Chapter 27, it is important to determine where the level of twist or torsion of the leg is and rule out tibial torsion or torsion of the foot.

This chapter provides various stretching and strengthening activities designed to decrease internal rotation of the hips and strengthen the external rotators of the hips. It is important for the treating therapist to focus on proper postural, hip, and foot alignment during these activities in order to achieve the desired goal.

DECREASING INTERNAL ROTATION OF THE HIPS

Positioning and Stretching Activities

- Tailor-sitting activities
  - Child tailor sits on floor.
  - Child sits in tailor-sitting position and plays catch with therapist.
  - Child sits in tailor-sitting position and reaches for items on both sides (Figures 28-1 and 28-2).
- Tailor stretching
  - Butterfly stretch: Child sits with back against wall and soles of feet touching. Child holds onto ankles and gently moves knees up and down, flapping them like butterflies.

Danto, A. H., & Pruzansky, M. *1001 Pediatric Treatment Activities: Creative Ideas for Therapy Sessions, Third Edition* (pp. 175-179).
© 2023 SLACK Incorporated.

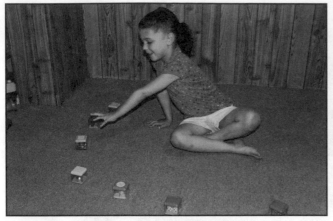

Figure 28-1.

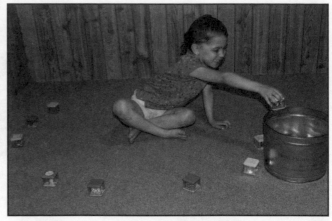

Figure 28-2.

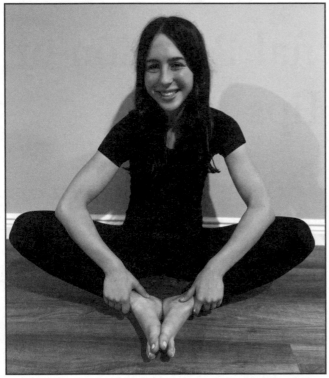

Figure 28-3.

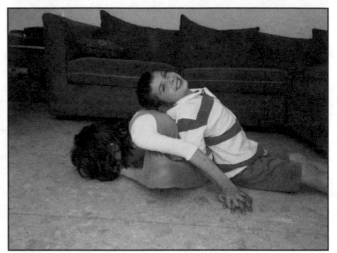

Figure 28-4.

- Duck-walking: Therapist instructs child to turn feet out and walk across room with feet turned out and quack like a duck.

- Therapist tapes cutout footprints onto floor with footprints externally rotated. Child walks along path, aligning feet to the footprints.

- Child stands with feet in neutral or externally rotated position and does the following:

  ○ Jumps in the air 10 times.

  ○ Jumps to pull Post-It Notes off the wall.

  ○ Jumps over cones in obstacle course.

- Ballet poses

  ○ Therapist teaches child first position (Figure 28-5).

  ○ Therapist teaches child second position (Figure 28-6).

  ○ Therapist teaches child third position (Figure 28-7).

○ Tailor press: Child sits with back against wall and soles of feet touching. Child holds onto ankles and gently presses down on knees with elbows (Figure 28-3).

○ Partner tailor stretch: Children sit back to back. Child 1 sits with soles of feet touching, holding ankles. Child 2 leans back into child 1 with appropriate pressure to stretch. Therapist supervises (Figure 28-4).

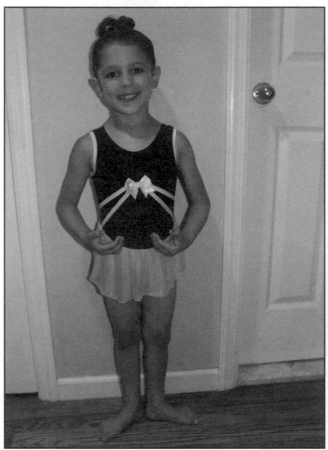

Figure 28-5.

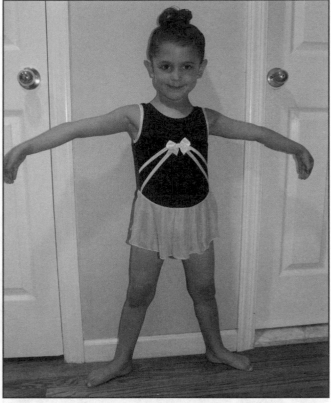

Figure 28-6.

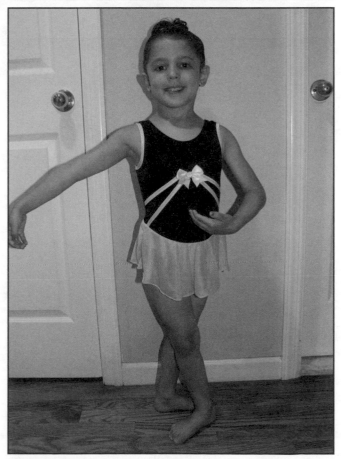

Figure 28-7.

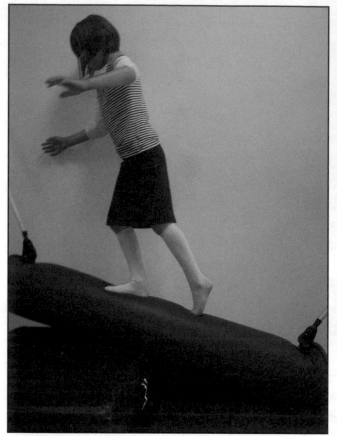

Figure 28-8.

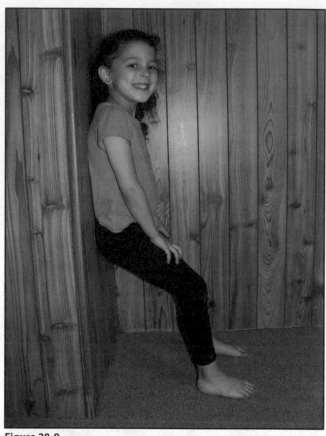

Figure 28-9.

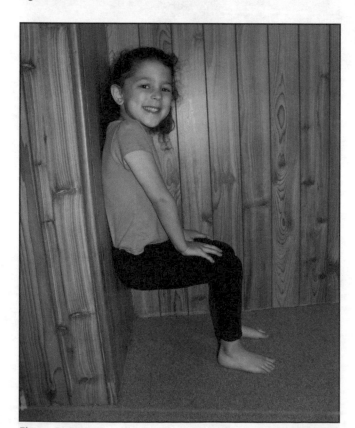

Figure 28-10.

Strengthening Activities

- Climbing activities
  - Child climbs up rope ladder.
  - Child climbs up bars on playground equipment or ladder.
  - Child climbs up rock wall.
- Therapist places bolster on incline against wall. Child walks up bolster slowly (Figure 28-8).
- Squatting activities
  - Isolated squats: Child performs set number of squats, maintaining proper hip alignment.
  - Child reaches down to pick object up off floor and place in a higher container.
  - Child leans against wall with hips in neutral and slowly lowers self through squat (Figures 28-9 and 28-10).

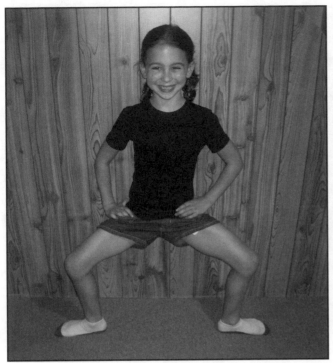

Figure 28-11.

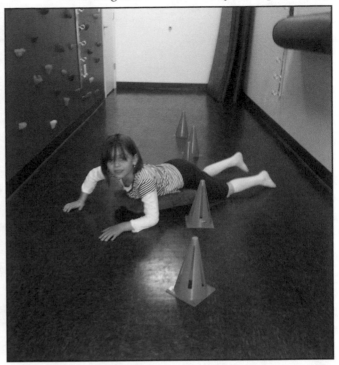

Figure 28-12.

○ Child leans against wall with hips externally rotated and slowly lowers self through squat (Figure 28-11).

○ Child sits on peanut-shaped therapy ball and completes squats.

Activities to Promote Having the Feet in a Neutral or Externally Rotated Position

- Prone scooter activities
  ○ Child propels self on scooter using only legs.
  ○ Child weaves through different cones in obstacle course while prone on scooter (Figure 28-12).

- Roller skating activities
  ○ Child skates in straight line across floor.
  ○ Child takes steps in roller skates.
  ○ Child moves right foot in clockwise circles on floor. Child then moves left foot in counterclockwise circles on floor.

- Therapist places small pieces of fabric or carpet squares on floor and child skates on them.

Addressing Toe-Walking

Toe-walking is a condition where children walk on the balls of their feet. It is sometimes seen in small children learning to walk; however, they will usually have a typical heel-to-toe gait by 3 years old (Jacobs, 2010).

Toe-walking can be the symptom of neurological influences, a result of trauma, or may have no known cause (i.e., idiopathic toe-walking; Williams et al., 2013). When children walk on their toes, it can cause pain in surrounding contracted muscles (Solan et al., 2010) and affect their ability to fully engage in age-appropriate activities (Engström & Tedroff, 2012).

Various treatment techniques have been developed to address toe-walking with varying degrees of success (Williams et al., 2013). It is important for the therapist to first identify the cause if possible. Once this is done, they can then select the appropriate course of treatment.

This chapter provides various stretching, strengthening, and sensory activities that help limit toe-walking in young children. In addition to these activities, various techniques developed by other medical professionals are sometimes employed, including serial casting, orthotics, and the use of medical injections of botulinum toxin (Williams et al., 2013). A trained physical or occupational therapist can help determine the proper course of treatment in treating a child who toe-walks as well as the need for other services.

ADDRESSING TOE-WALKING

Activities Promoting Flat Foot Placement

- Heavy pushing: Child pushes heavy cart or object across floor.
- Child pushes walking toys across room (Figure 29-1).
- Stepping activities
  - Child stands on a raised surface or crate and slowly lowers one leg at a time to the ground (opposite leg will get stretched; Figure 29-2).
  - Child stands in front of crate and raises one leg up onto crate backward to step onto crate. Raised leg will get stretched (Figure 29-3).
  - Child descends flight of stairs, alternating feet if possible.
  - Child ascends flight of stairs backward with close supervision.

Danto, A. H., & Pruzansky, M. *1001 Pediatric Treatment Activities: Creative Ideas for Therapy Sessions, Third Edition* (pp. 181-186).
© 2023 SLACK Incorporated.

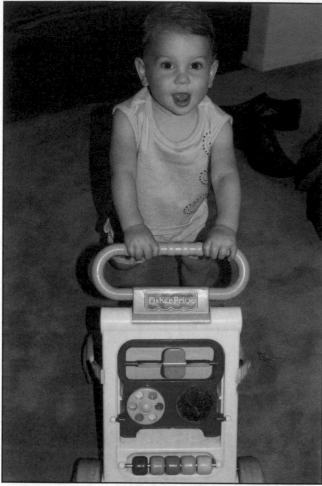

Figure 29-1.

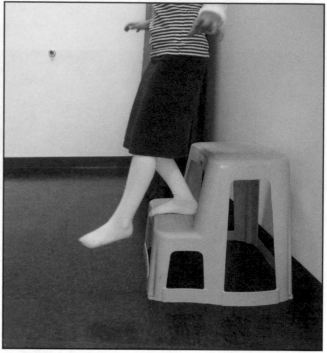

Figure 29-2.

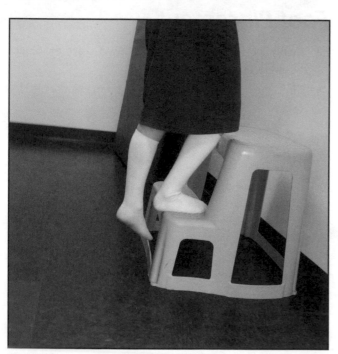

Figure 29-3.

- Therapist places hands on child's shoulder giving input for child to keep toes flat on ground. Child walks across room, with therapist maintaining gentle physical input down and onto child's shoulders (Figure 29-4).

- Standing on unstable surfaces
  - Child stands on large pillow barefoot and reaches one at a time for multiple items scattered around the pillow on floor.
  - Child stands on Dynadisc with bare feet and balances for several seconds.
  - Child walks across large bean bags placed on floor.
  - Child stands on balance board while completing puzzle placed on floor in front of balance board.

- Roller skating activities
  - Child skates in straight line across floor.
  - Child skates backward while holding therapists hands, focusing on pressing feet into floor.
  - Child takes steps in roller skates.

- Scooter activities
  - Child sits on scooter and pulls self forward across room, focusing on pulling self with heels.

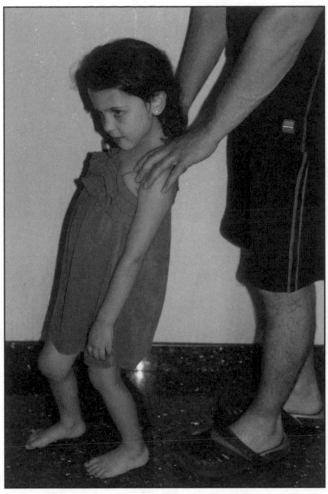

Figure 29-4.

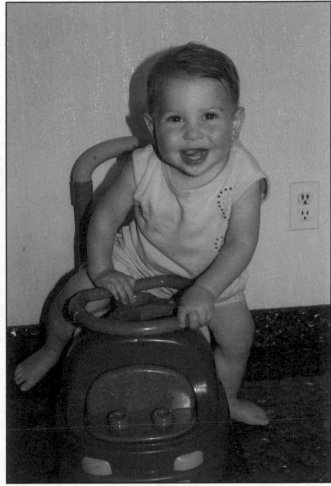

Figure 29-5.

- Child sits on scooter and pushes self backward across room, focusing on keeping feet flat on floor when pushing.
- Activities with riding toys (Figures 29-5 and 29-6)
  - Child sits on riding toy and pulls self forward across room, focusing on pulling self with heels.
  - Child sits on riding toy and pushes self backward across room, focusing on keeping feet flat on floor when pushing.
- Child sits on top of large plush toy and uses feet to pull self around room (Figure 29-7).

- Child steps firmly on stepping stones and presses them into floor.
- Child steps backward up a ramp.
- Child walks forward up a ramp.
- Child walks on treadmill on increased incline with direct therapist supervision.
- Child frog-hops across room.
- Child bear-walks across room.

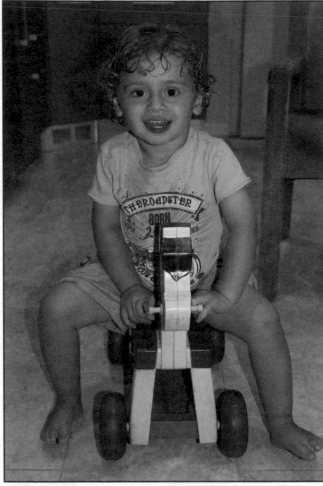

Figure 29-6.

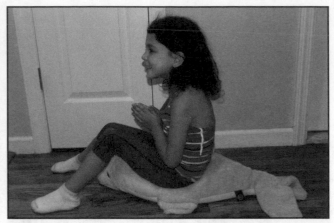

Figure 29-7.

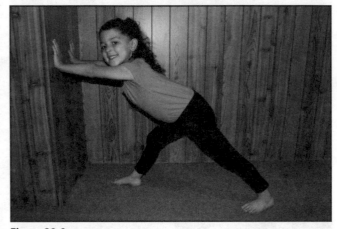

Figure 29-9.

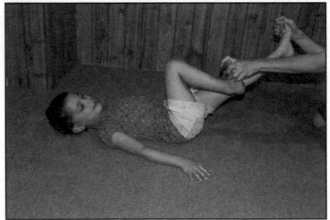

Figure 29-8.

Stretching Exercises

- Child lies on back and therapist moves child's feet in bicycle position (Figure 29-8).
- Child pushes against wall with one leg in front of the other and back leg straight (Figure 29-9).

- Child places one foot on curb and one foot on floor and bends down to touch curb (Figure 29-10).

(These should always be followed by meaningful activities.)

Sensory Activities Providing Input to Bottoms of Feet

- Child walks barefoot along floor on various textures, concentrating on keeping feet flat.
- Child stands in rice box.
- Child walks across sand box.
- Child jumps barefoot on trampoline.
- Child walks across mushy bean bags placed on floor.
- Child walks across room with ankle weights.
- Child walks while wearing weighted vest or with weighted blanket on shoulders.
- Child wears high-top sneakers and walks across room.

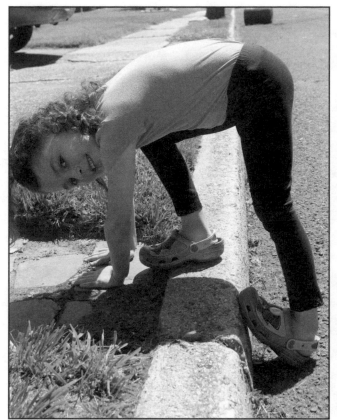

Figure 29-10.

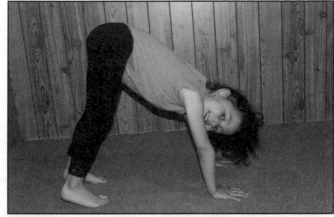

Figure 29-11.

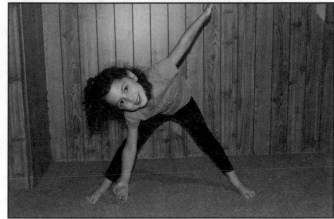

Figure 29-13.

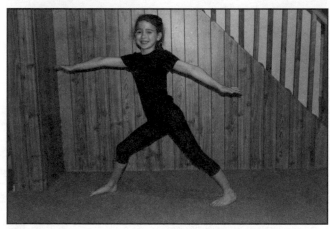

Figure 29-12.

Yoga Positions

- Downward dog (Figure 29-11)
- Warrior position (Figure 29-12)
- Triangle pose (Figure 29-13)
- Forward fold (Figure 29-14)
- Forward fold with a partner (Figure 29-15)

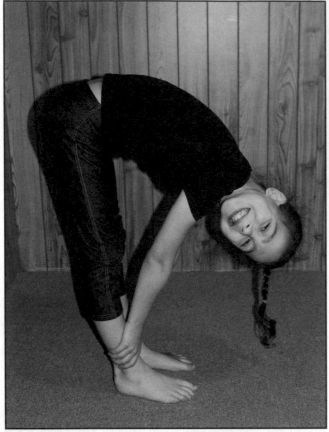

Figure 29-14.

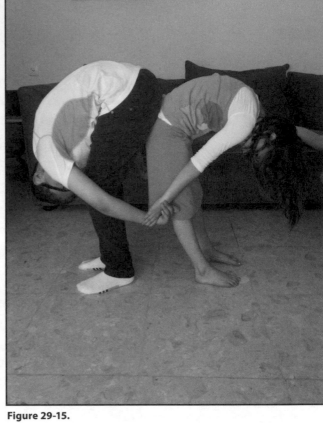

Figure 29-15.

References

Alaniz, M. L., Galit, E., Necesito, C. I., & Rosario, E. R. (2015). Hand strength, handwriting, and functional skills in children with autism. *American Journal of Occupational Therapy, 69*(4), 6904220030p1-6904220030p9.

Alston, J., & Taylor, J. (1987). *Handwriting: Theory, research, and practice.* Nichols.

Andreasen, J., Mølgaard, C. M., Christensen, M., Kaalundb, S., Lundbye-Christensen, S., Simonsen, O., & Voigte, M. (2013). Exercise therapy and custom-made insoles are effective in patients with excessive pronation and chronic foot pain—a randomized controlled trial. *The Foot, 23,* 22-28.

Axelsson, I., Holmblad, A., & Johansson, J. (2019). Restoring visual capacity after stroke using an intense office-based vision therapy program: Three case reports. *Clinical Case Reports, 7*(4), 707-713.

Ayres, A. J. (1965). Patterns of perceptual-motor dysfunction in children: A factor analytic study. *Perceptual and Motor Skills, 20,* 355-368.

Ayres, A. J. (1972). *Sensory integration and learning disorders.* Western Psychological Services.

Ayres, A. J. (1979). *Sensory integration and the child.* Western Psychological Services.

Ayres, A. J. (2005). *Sensory integration and the child. Understanding hidden sensory challenges.* Western Psychological Service.

Baranek, G. T. (2002). Efficacy of sensory and motor interventions for children with autism. *Journal of Autism and Developmental Disorders, 32*(5), 397-422.

Bart, O., Hajami, D., & Bar-Haim, Y. (2007). Predicting school adjustment from motor abilities in kindergarten. *Infant and Child Development, 16*(6), 597-615. https://psycnet.apa.org/doi/10.1002/icd.514

Bazyk, S., Michaud, P., Goodman, G., Papp, P., Hawkins, E., & Welch, M. A. (2009). Integrating occupational therapy services in a kindergarten curriculum: A look at the outcomes. *American Journal of Occupational Therapy, 63*(2), 160-171.

Beery, K. E. (2004). *The Beery-Buktenica developmental test of visual-motor integration* (5th ed.). NCS Pearson, Inc.

Beery, K. E., Buktenica, N. A., & Beery, N. A. (2010). *The Beery-Buktenica developmental test of visual-motor integration* (6th ed.). Pearson.

Benbow, M. (1995). Principles and practices of teaching handwriting. In A. Henderson & C. Pehoski (Eds.), *Hand function in the child: Foundations for remediation* (pp. 255-281). Mosby-Year Book.

Benbow, M. (1997). *A neurokinesthetic approach to hand function and handwriting.* Advanced Rehabilitation Institutes.

Ben-Yishay, Y., Piasetsky, E. B., & Rattok, J. (1987). A systematic method for ameliorating disorders in basic attention. In M. J. Meier, A. L. Benton, & L. Diller (Eds.), *Neuropsychological rehabilitation* (pp. 165-181). The Guilford Press.

Bertani, A., Cappello, A., Benedetti, M. G., Simoncini, L., & Catani, F. (1999). Flat foot functional evaluation using pattern recognition of ground reaction data. *Clinical Biomechanics, 14*(7), 484-493.

Biederman, J., Monuteaux, M. C., Doyle, A. E., Seidman, L. J., Wilens, T. E., Ferrero, F., & Faraone, S. V. (2004). Impact of executive function deficits and attention-deficit/hyperactivity disorder (ADHD) on academic outcomes in children. *Journal of Consulting and Clinical Psychology, 72*(5), 757-766.

Blakemore, S. J., Tavassoli, T., Calò, S., Thomas, R. M., Catmur, C., Frith, U., & Haggard, P. (2006). Tactile sensitivity in Asperger syndrome. *Brain and Cognition, 61*(1), 5-13.

Blanche, E. I., Reinoso, G., Chang, M. C., & Bodison, S. (2012). Proprioceptive processing difficulties among children with autism spectrum disorders and developmental disabilities. *American Journal of Occupational Therapy, 66*(5), 621-624.

Burnett, R., Cornett, N., Rekart, G., Donahoe-Fillmore, B., Brahler, C. J., Aebker, S., & Kreill, M. (2011). Investigating the associations between core strength, postural control and fine motor performance in children. *Journal of Student Physical Therapy Research, 4*(2), 40-47.

Carbone, V. J., O'Brien, L., Sweeney-Kerwin, E. J., & Albert, K. M. (2013). Teaching eye contact to children with autism: A conceptual analysis and single case study. *Education and Treatment of Children, 36*(2), 139-159.

Cardona, M. D. P., Martinez, A. L., & Hinojosa, J. (2000). Effectiveness of using a computer to improve attention to visual analysis activities of five preschool children with disabilities. *Occupational Therapy International, 7*(1), 42-56.

Case-Smith, J. (2001). *Occupational therapy for children.* Mosby, Inc.

Danto, A. H., & Pruzansky, M. 1001 *Pediatric Treatment Activities: Creative Ideas for Therapy Sessions, Third Edition* (pp. 187-190).
© 2023 SLACK Incorporated.

Cermak, S. A., Quintero, E. J., & Cohen, P. M. (1980). Developmental age trends in crossing the body midline in normal children. *American Journal of Occupational Therapy, 34*(5), 313-319.

Cheldavi, H., Shakerian, S., Boshehri, S. N. S., & Zarghami, M. (2014). The effects of balance training intervention on postural control of children with autism spectrum disorder: Role of sensory information. *Research in Autism Spectrum Disorders, 8*(1), 8-14.

Chen, S. T., Sultzer, D. L., Hinkin, C. H., Mahler, M. E., & Cummings, J. L. (1998). Executive dysfunction in Alzheimer's disease: Association with neuropsychiatric symptoms and functional impairment. *The Journal of Neuropsychiatry and Clinical Neurosciences, 10*(4), 426-432.

Cibulka, M. T., Strube, M. J., Meier, D., Selsor, M., Wheatley, C., Wilson, N. G., & Irrgang, J. J. (2010). Symmetrical and asymmetrical hip rotation and its relationship to hip rotator muscle strength. *Clinical Biomechanics, 25*(1), 56-62.

Cohen, H. (1992). Vestibular rehabilitation reduces functional disability. *Otolaryngology—Head and Neck Surgery, 107*(5), 638-643.

Combs, M. L., & Slaby, D. A. (1977). Social-skills training with children. In B. B. Lahey & A. E. Kazdin (Eds.), *Advances in clinical child psychology* (pp. 161-201). Springer.

Cooke, D. M., McKenna, K., & Fleming, J. (2005). Development of a standardized occupational therapy screening tool for visual perception in adults. *Scandinavian Journal of Occupational Therapy, 12*(2), 59-71.

Cornhill, H., & Case-Smith, J. (1996). Factors that relate to good and poor handwriting. *American Journal of Occupational Therapy, 50*, 732-739.

Cottrell, R. P. F. (2004). *National occupational therapy certification exam review & study guide.* International Education Resources.

Cowen, E. L., Pederson, A., Babigian, H., Isso, L. D., & Trost, M. A. (1973). Long-term follow-up of early detected vulnerable children. *Journal of Consulting and Clinical Psychology, 41*(3), 438-446.

Daly, C. J., Kelley, G. T., & Krauss, A. (2003). Relationship between visual-motor integration and handwriting skills of children in kindergarten: A modified replication study. *American Journal of Occupational Therapy, 57*(4), 459-462.

Davich, J. A. (2005). *A comparison of interventions for children with tactile defensiveness* [Master's thesis, University of Wisconsin-Stout]. MINDS@UW. https://minds.wisconsin.edu/bitstream/handle/1793/41587/2005davichj.pdf?sequence=1&isAllowed=y

DeGangi, G. A. (1994). *Documenting sensorimotor progress: a pediatric therapist's guide.* Therapy Skill Builders.

Diekema, S. M., Deitz, J., & Amundson, S. J. (1998). Test–retest reliability of the Evaluation Tool of Children's Handwriting-Manuscript. *American Journal of Occupational Therapy, 52*(4), 248-255.

Dunbar, S. B. (1999). A child's occupational performance: Considerations of sensory processing and family context. *American Journal of Occupational Therapy, 53*(2), 231-235.

Dunn, W. (2001). The 2001 Eleanor Clarke Slagle Lecture. The sensations of everyday life: Empirical, theoretical, and pragmatic considerations. *American Journal of Occupational Therapy, 55*(6), 608-620.

DuPaul, G. J., & Stoner, G. (2014). *ADHD in the schools: Assessment and intervention strategies.* Guilford Publications.

Effgen, K. (2005). Child development and appraisal. In K. Effgen (Ed.), *Meeting the physical therapy needs of children* (pp. 74-75). F. A. Davis Company.

Engström, P., & Tedroff, K. (2012). The prevalence and course of idiopathic toe-walking in 5-year-old children. *Pediatrics, 130*(2), 279-284.

Exner, C. E. (1997). Clinical interpretation of "In-hand manipulation in young children: Translation movements." *American Journal of Occupational Therapy, 51*(9), 729-732.

Farris, K., Fehrenbacher, R., Hayes, E., McEvoy, R., Smith, A., & McCulloch, R. (2019). The relationship between muscle activation and handwriting quality with different grip styles. *International Journal of Exercise Science: Conference Proceedings, 8*(7), 57.

Foster, S. M., & Verny, T. R. (2007). The development of sensory systems during the prenatal period. *Journal of Prenatal & Perinatal Psychology & Health, 21*(3), 271-280.

Gerber, R. J., Wilks, T., & Erdie-Lalena, C. (2010). Developmental milestones: Motor development. *Pediatrics in Review, 31*(7), 267-277.

Giroux Bruce, M. A., & Borg, B. (2002). *Psychosocial frames of reference.* SLACK Incorporated.

Granacher, U., Gollhofer, A., Hortobágyi, T., Kressig, R. W., & Muehlbauer, T. (2013). The importance of trunk muscle strength for balance, functional performance, and fall prevention in seniors: A systematic review. *Sports Medicine, 43*(7), 627-641.

Granacher, U., Gollhofer, A., & Kriemler, S. (2010). Effects of balance training on postural sway, leg extensor strength, and jumping height in adolescents. *Research Quarterly for Exercise and Sport, 81*(3), 245-251.

Grandin, T. (1992). Calming effects of deep touch pressure in patients with autistic disorder, college students, and animals. *Journal of Child and Adolescent Psychopharmacology, 2*(1), 63-72.

Häger-Ross, C., & Rösblad, B. (2002). Norms for grip strength in children aged 4–16 years. *Acta Paediatrica, 91*(6), 617-625.

Harris, T. L., & Rarick, G. L. (1959). The relationship between handwriting pressure and legibility of handwriting in children and adolescents. *The Journal of Experimental Education, 28*(1), 65-84.

Hervey-Jumper, S. L., Justice, D., Vanaman, M. M., Nelson, V. S., & Yang, L. J. S. (2011). Torticollis associated with neonatal brachial plexus palsy. *Pediatric Neurology, 45*(5), 305-310.

Hochreiter, N. W., Jewell, M. J., Barber, L., & Browne, P. (1983). Effect of vibration on tactile sensitivity. *Physical Therapy, 63*(6), 934-937.

Horak, F. B., Jones-Rycewicz, C., Black, F. O., & Shumway-Cook, A. (1992). Effects of vestibular rehabilitation on dizziness and imbalance. *Otolaryngology–Head and Neck Surgery, 106*(2), 175-180.

Huffman, J. M., & Fortenberry, C. (2011). Developing fine motor skills. *Young Children, 66*(5), 100-103.

Jacini, W. F., Cannonieri, G. C., Fernandes, P. T., Bonilha, L., Cendes, F., & Li, L. M. (2009). Can exercise shape your brain? Cortical differences associated with judo practice. *Journal of Science and Medicine in Sport, 12*(6), 688-690.

Jacobs, B. (2010). Toe walking, flat feet and bow legs, in-toeing and out-toeing. *Paediatrics and Child Health, 20*, 221-224.

Jeffreys, I. (2002). Developing a progressive core stability program. *Strength & Conditioning Journal, 24*(5), 65-66.

Jones, L. A., & Lederman, S. J. (2006). *Human hand function* (1st ed.). Oxford University Press.

Jones, S. M., Jones, T. A., Mills, K. N., & Gaines, G. C. (2009). Anatomical and physiological considerations in vestibular dysfunction and compensation. *Seminars in Hearing, 30*(4), 231-241.

Kavale, K. (1982). Meta-analysis of the relationship between visual perceptual skills and reading achievement. *Journal of Learning Disabilities, 15*(1), 42-51.

Koziol, L. F., Budding, D. E., & Chidekel, D. (2011). Sensory integration, sensory processing, and sensory modulation disorders: Putative functional neuroanatomic underpinnings. *The Cerebellum, 10*(4), 770-792.

Kumin, L., Von Hagel, K. C., & Bahr, D. C. (2001). An effective oral motor intervention protocol for infants and toddlers with low muscle tone. *Infant Toddler Intervention, 11*(3/4), 181-200.

Kwon, J. Y., & Myerson, M. S. (2010). Management of the flexible foot in the child: A focus on the use of osteotomies for corrections. *The Pediatric Foot and Ankle, 15*(2), 309-322.

Langberg, J. M., Epstein, J. N., & Graham, A. J. (2008). Organizational-skills interventions in the treatment of ADHD. *Expert Review of Neurotherapeutics, 8*(10), 1549-1561.

Lemon, R. N., Mantel, G. W., & Muir, R. B. (1986). Corticospinal facilitation of hand muscles during voluntary movement in the conscious monkey. *The Journal of Physiology, 381*(1), 497-527.

Losse, A., Henderson, S. E., Elliman, D., Hall, D., Knight, E., & Jongmans, M. (1991). Clumsiness in children-do they grow out of it? A 10-year follow-up study. *Developmental Medicine & Child Neurology, 33*(1), 55-68.

Markowitz, M. (2006). Occupational therapy interventions in low vision rehabilitation. *Canadian Journal of Ophthalmology, 41*(3), 340-347.

Marr, D., Cermak, S., Cohn, E. S., & Henderson, A. (2003). Fine motor activities in Head Start and kindergarten classrooms. *American Journal of Occupational Therapy, 57*(5), 550-557.

Martin, N. A. (2006). *Test of visual perceptual skills—non motor* (3rd ed.). Academic Therapy Publications.

Michelson, L., Sugai, D. P., Wood, R. P., & Kazdin, A. E. (2013). *Social skills assessment and training with children: An empirically based handbook.* Springer Science & Business Media.

Miller, A., Moncayo, Z., Treadwell, D., & Olson, L. (1999, April).*Children with autism using weighted vests: Two single-subject studies* [Paper presentation]. The American Occupational Therapy Association Annual Conference and Exposition, Indianapolis, Indiana.

Miller, L. J., Anzalone, M. E., Lane, S. J., Cermak, S. A., & Osten, E. T. (2007). Concept evolution in sensory integration: A proposed nosology for diagnosis. *American Journal of Occupational Therapy, 61*(2), 135-140.

Müller, S., Carlsohn, A., Müller, J., Heiner, B., & Mayer, F. (2012). Static and dynamic foot characteristics in children aged 1–13 years: a cross-sectional study. *Gait & Posture, 35,* 389-394.

Muttiah, N., Georges, K., & Brackenbury, T. (2011). Clinical and research perspectives on nonspeech oral motor treatments and evidence-based practice. *American Journal of Speech-Language Pathology, 20*(1), 47-59.

Nederkoorn, C., Jansen, A., & Havermans, R. C. (2015). Feel your food. The influence of tactile sensitivity on picky eating in children. *Appetite, 84,* 7-10.

Oliver, C. E. (1990). A sensorimotor program for improving writing readiness skills in elementary-age children. *American Journal of Occupational Therapy, 44,* 111-116.

Parham, D. L., & Fazio, L. S. (1997). *Play in occupational therapy for children.* Mosby, Inc.

Parush, S., Yochman, A., Cohen, D., & Gershon, E. (1998). Relation of visual perception and visual-motor integration for clumsy children. *Perceptual and Motor Skills, 86*(1), 291-295.

Pfeiffer, B., & Kinnealey, M. (2003). Treatment of sensory defensiveness in adults. *Occupational Therapy International, 10*(3), 175-184.

Piek, J. P., Baynam, G. B., & Barrett, N. C. (2006). The relationship between fine and gross motor ability, self-perceptions and self-worth in children and adolescents. *Human Movement Science, 25*(1), 65-75.

Rachwani, J., Santamaria, V., Saavedra, S. L., & Woollacott, M. H. (2015). The development of trunk control and its relation to reaching in infancy: A longitudinal study. *Frontiers in Human Neuroscience, 9,* 94.

Raghavan, P., Krakauer, J., Santello, M., & Gordon, A. (2007). Relationship between finger individuation and shaping the fingers to object contours. *American Journal of Physical Medicine & Rehabilitation, 86*(4), 327.

Reichow, B., Barton, E., Neely Sewell, J., Good, L., & Wolery, M. (2010). Effects of weighted vests on the engagement of children with developmental delays and autism. *Focus on Autism and Other Developmental Disabilities, 25*(1), 3-11.

Reisman, J. E. (1991). Poor handwriting: Who is referred? *American Journal of Occupational Therapy, 45,*849-852.

Rine, R. M. (2009). Growing evidence for balance and vestibular problems in children. *Audiological Medicine, 7*(3), 138-142.

Rine, R. M., & Wiener-Vacher, S. (2013). Evaluation and treatment of vestibular dysfunction in children. *NeuroRehabilitation, 32*(3), 507-518.

Robinson, D. A. (1968). The oculomotor control system: A review. *Proceedings of the IEEE, 56*(6), 1032-1049.

Rosenfeld-Johnson, S. (2001). *Oral-motor exercises for speech clarity.* Innovative Therapists International.

Salar, S., Daneshmandi, H., Karimizadeh Ardakani, M., & Nazari Sharif, H. (2014). The relationship of core strength with static and dynamic balance in children with autism. *Annals of Applied Sport Science, 2*(4), 33-42.

Schaft, R., & Roley, S. (2006). *Sensory integration: Applying clinical reasoning to practice with diverse population* (pp. 52, 74-80).

Schmidt, A., Dirk, J., & Schmiedek, F. (2019). The importance of peer relatedness at school for affective well-being in children: Between- and within-person associations. *Social Development, 28*(4), 873-892.

Schneck, C. M. (1996). Visual perception. *Occupational Therapy for Children* (6th ed., pp. 373-403). Mosby, Inc.

Shumway-Cook, A., Hutchinson, S., Kartin, D., Price, R., & Woollacott, M. (2003). Effect of balance training on recovery of stability in children with cerebral palsy. *Developmental Medicine & Child Neurology, 45*(9), 591-602.

Shumway-Cook, A., & Woollacott, M. H. (1995). *Motor control: Theory and practical applications.* Williams & Wilkins.

Silva, L., & Schalock, M. (2013). Treatment of tactile impairment in young children with autism: Results with qigong massage. *International Journal of Therapeutic Massage & Bodywork, 6*(4), 12-20.

Solan, M. C., Kohls-Gatzoulis, J., & Stephens, M. M. (2010). Idiopathic toe walking and contractures of the triceps surae. *The Pediatric Foot and Ankle, 15*(2), 297-307.

Srivastava, A. (2016). Sensory integration strategies for handwriting among autistic children. *Academic Journal of Pediatrics & Neonatology, 2*(1), 1-4.

Takata, N. (1974). Play as a prescription. In M. Reilly (Ed.), *Play as exploratory learning* (pp. 209-246). Sage Publications.

Tecklin, J. S. (2008). *Pediatric physical therapy* (4th ed.). Lippincott Williams & Wilkins.

Thielbar, K. O., Lord, T. J., Fischer, H. C., Lazzaro, E. C., Barth, K. C., Stoykov, M. E., & Kamper, D. G. (2014). Training finger individuation with a mechatronic-virtual reality system leads to improved fine motor control post-stroke. *Journal of Neuroengineering and Rehabilitation, 11*(1), 171.

Tudor, M. (1981). *Child development.* McGraw-Hill.

VandenBerg, N. L. (2001). The use of a weighted vest to increase on-task behavior in children with attention difficulties. *American Journal of Occupational Therapy, 55,* 621-628.

Van Hof, P., Van der Kamp, J., & Savelsbergh, G. J. P. (2002). The relation of unimanual and bimanual reaching to crossing the midline. *Child Development, 73,* 1353-1362.

Vygotsky, L. (1986). *Thought and language.* (Rev. ed.). Massachusetts Institute of Technology.

Wallen, M., & Walker, R. (1995). Occupational therapy practice with children with perceptual motor dysfunction: Findings of a literature review and survey. *Australian Occupational Therapy Journal, 42,* 15-25.

Welsh, M. C., & Pennington, B. F. (1988). Assessing frontal lobe functioning in children: Views from developmental psychology. *Developmental Neuropsychology, 4*(3), 199-230.

Wikipedia. (2020). Pangram. https://en.wikipedia.org/wiki/Pangram#cite_note-2

Wilbarger, P., & Wilbarger, J. (1991). *Sensory defensiveness in children aged 2–12: An intervention guide for parents and other caretakers.* Avanti Educational Programs.

Wilson, B. N., Kaplan, B. J., Crawford, S. G., Campbell, A., & Dewey, D. (2000). Reliability and validity of a parent questionnaire on childhood motor skills. *American Journal of Occupational Therapy, 54*(5), 484-493.

Williams, C. M., Michalitsis, J., Murphy, A., Rawicki, B., & Haines, T. P. (2013). Do external stimuli impact the gait of children with idiopathic toe walking? A study protocol for a within-subject randomised control trial. *Journal of Foot and Ankle Research, 3*(3), e002389.

Williamson, G. G., & Dorman, W. J. (2002). *Promoting social competence.* Hammill Institute on Disabilities.

190   References

Wong, A. L., Haith, A. M., & Krakauer, J. W. (2015). Motor planning. *The Neuroscientist, 21*(4), 385-398.

The Word Play Website. (2020). Some well-known pangrams. http://www.fun-with-words.com/pang_example.html

Wren, T. A. L., Rethlefsen, S., & Kay, R. M. (2005). Prevalence of specific gait abnormalities in children with cerebral palsy. *Journal of Pediatric Orthopaedics, 25,* 79-83.

Your Dictionary. (2020). Examples of pangrams. https://examples.yourdictionary.com/reference/examples/examples-of-pangrams.html

Zeigler-Dendy, C. A. (2002, February). Five components of executive function and a bird's-eye view of life with ADD and ADHD: Advice from young survivors. *CHADD Attention Magazine.* https://chadd.org/attention-magazine/attention-magazine-february-2002/

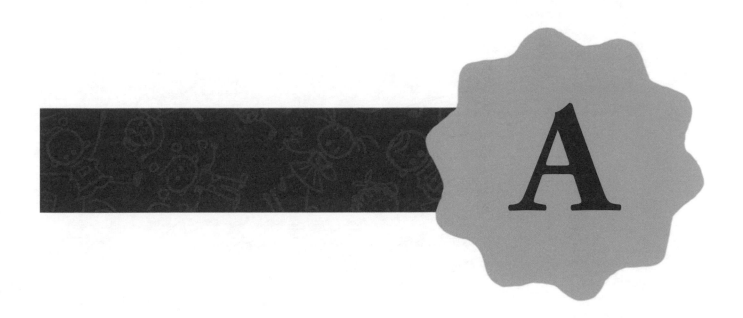

Worksheets and Handouts

Danto, A. H., & Pruzansky, M. *1001 Pediatric Treatment Activities:*
Creative Ideas for Therapy Sessions, Third Edition (pp. 191-254).
© 2023 SLACK Incorporated.

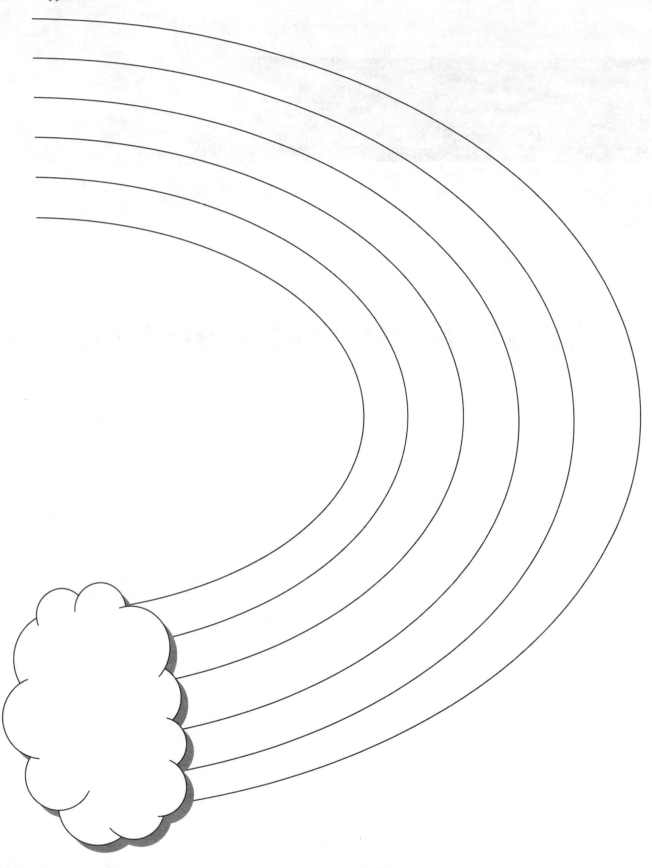

Cut out the boxes and then sort the following shapes from biggest to smallest

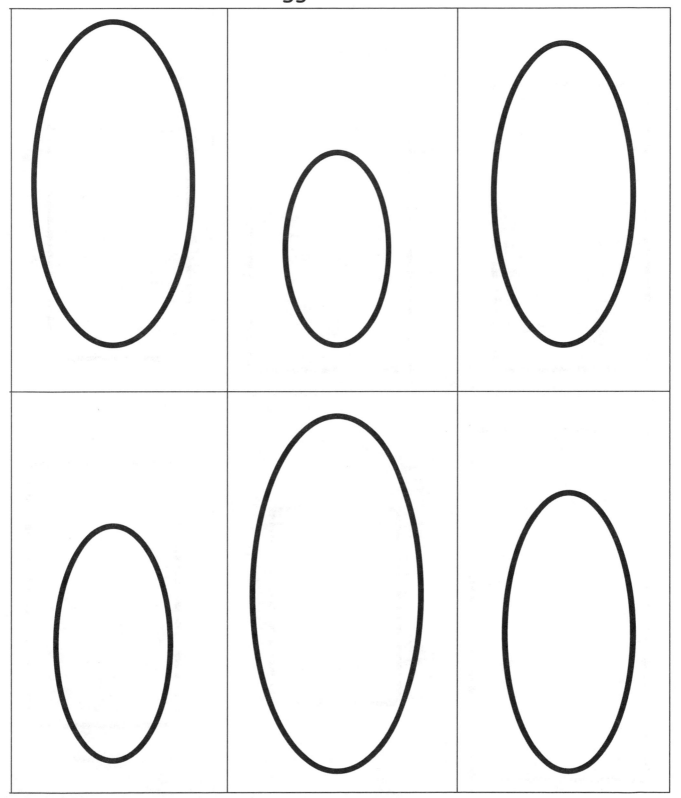

Cut out the boxes and then sort the following shapes from biggest to smallest

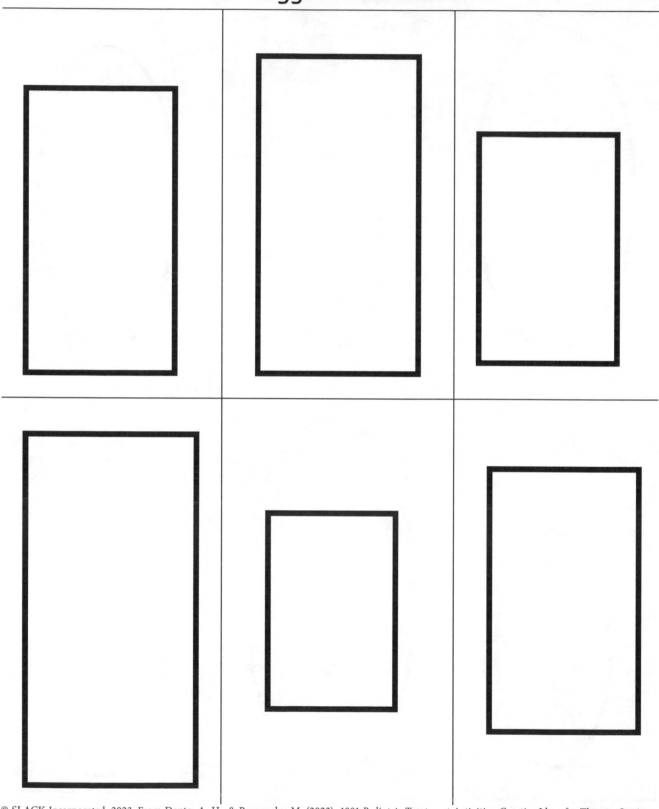

Cut out the boxes and then sort the following shapes from biggest to smallest

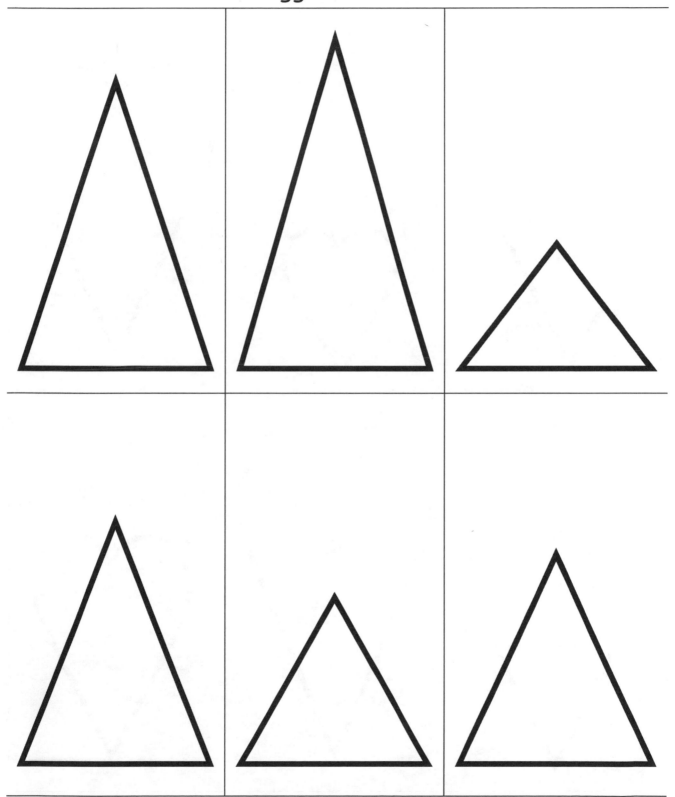

Cut out the boxes and then sort the following shapes from biggest to smallest

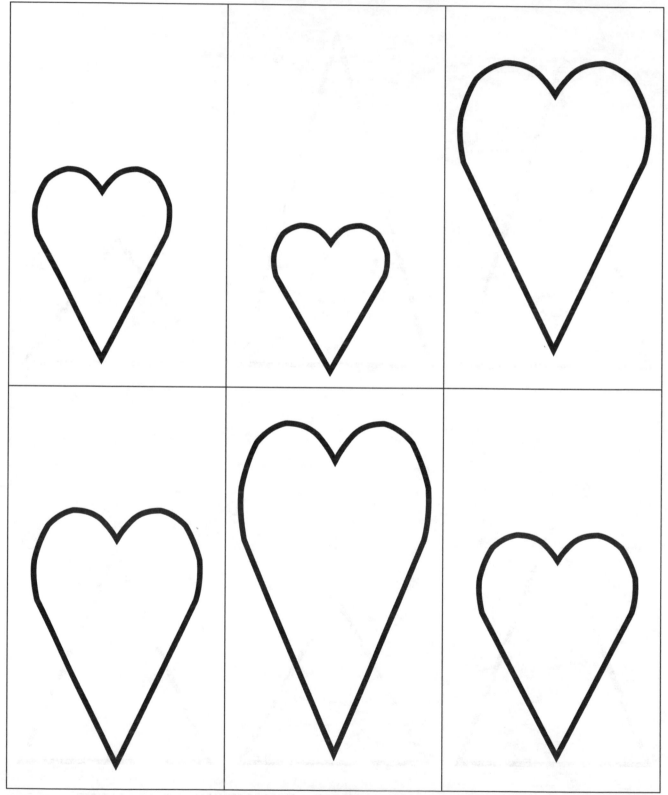

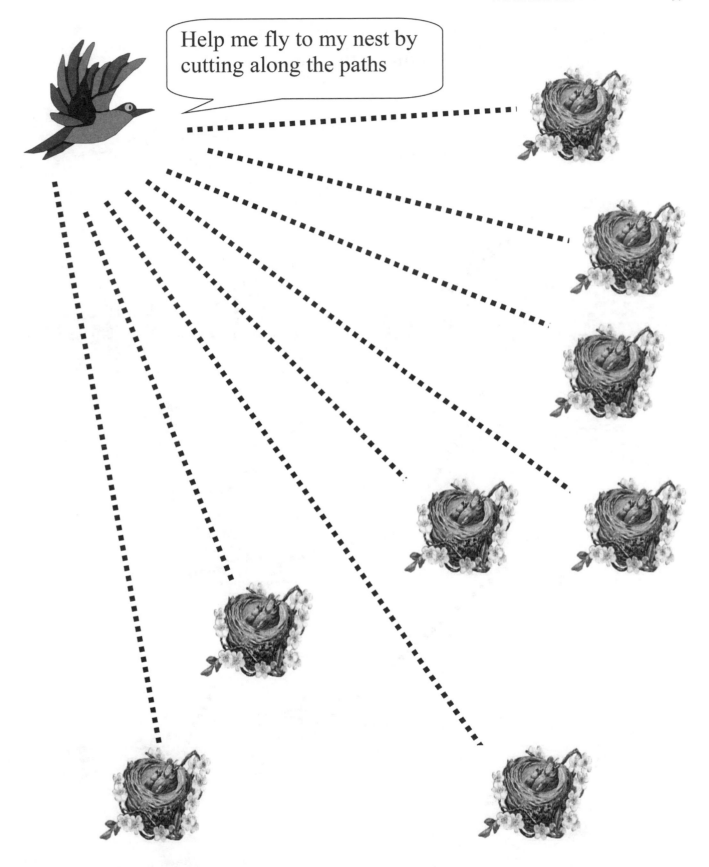

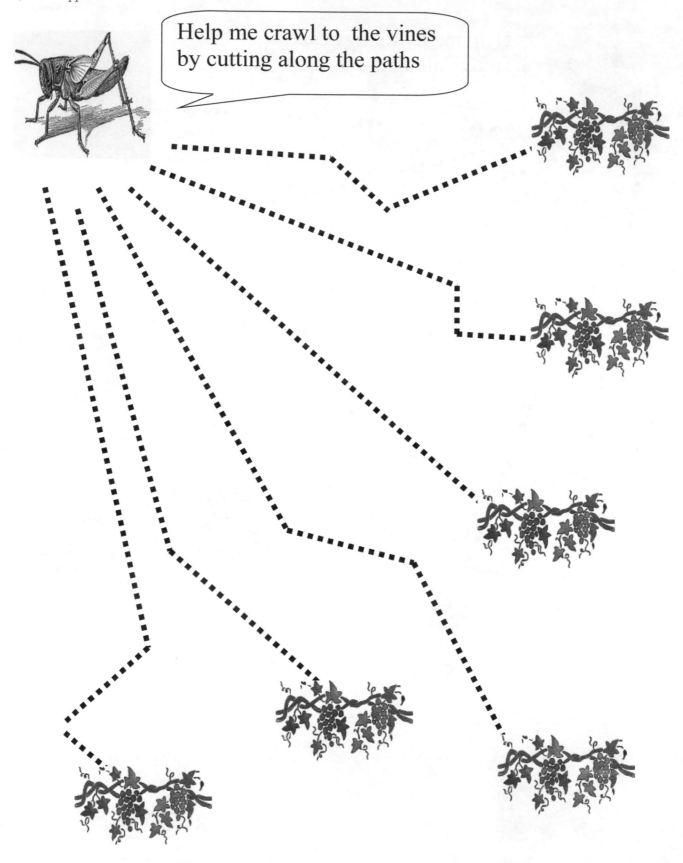

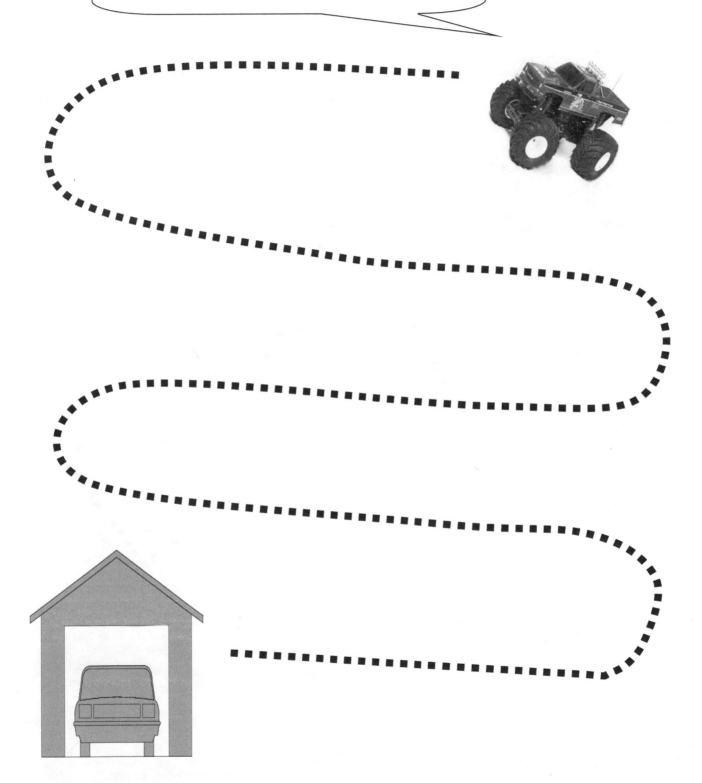

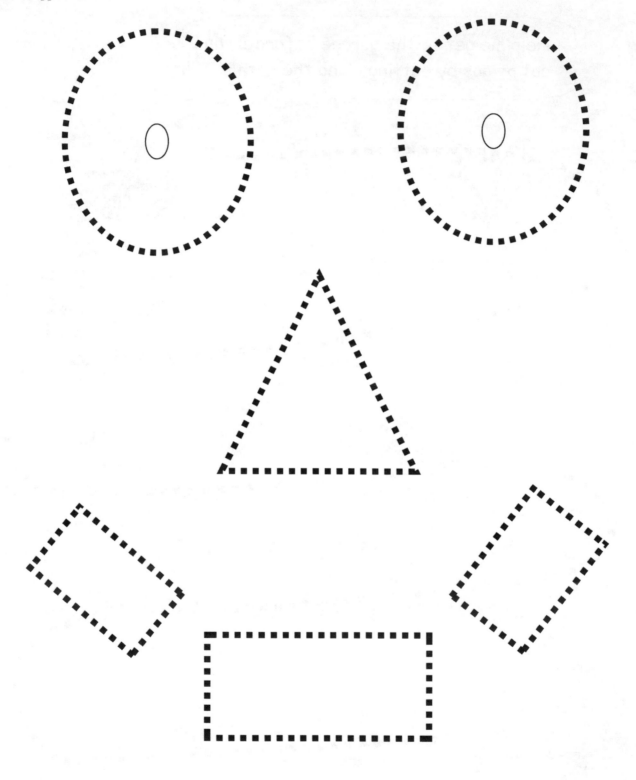

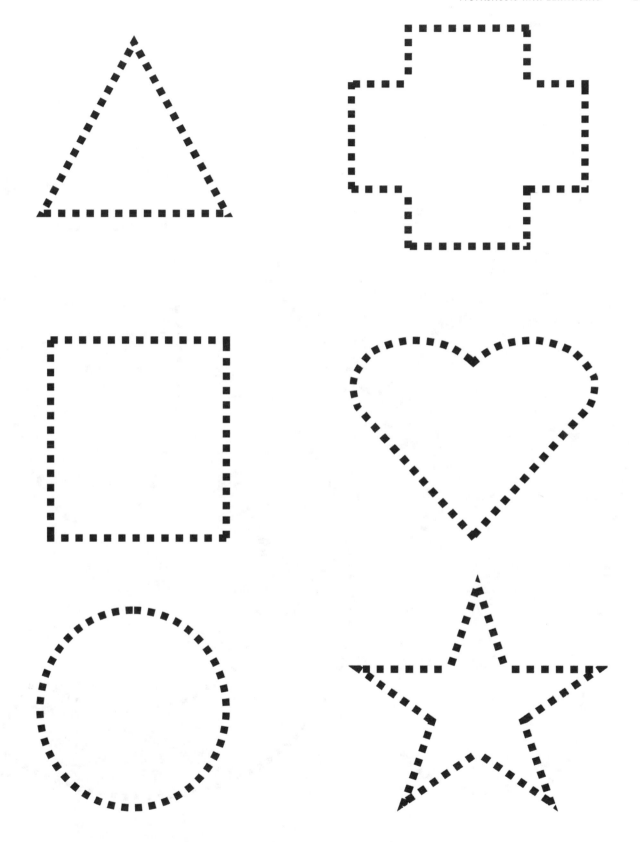

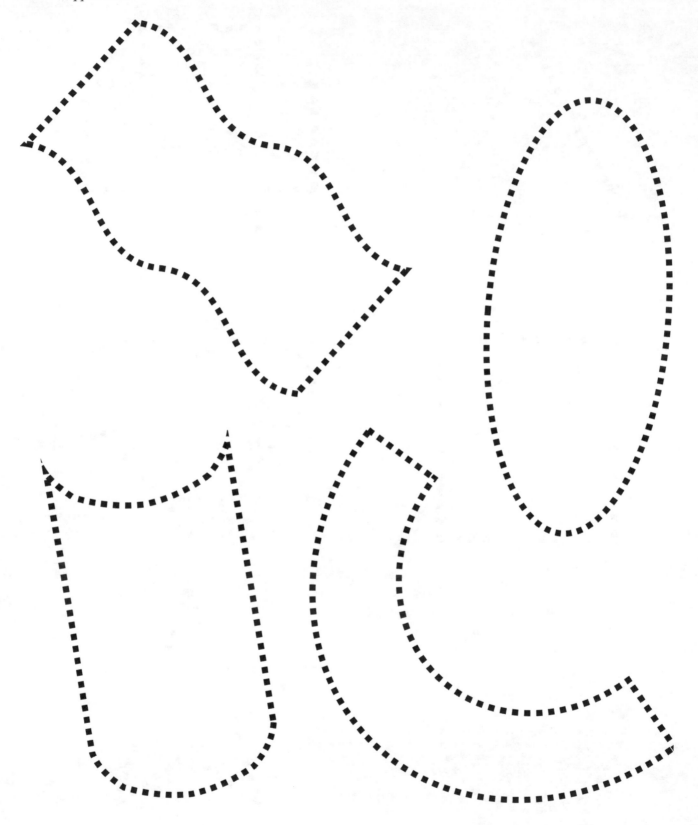

Which picture is different from the others?

1

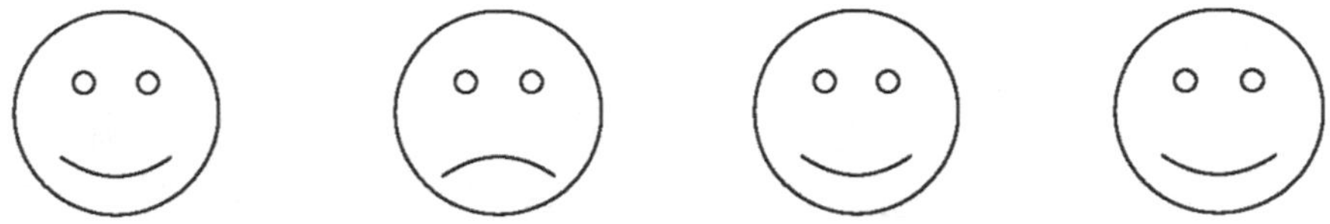

2

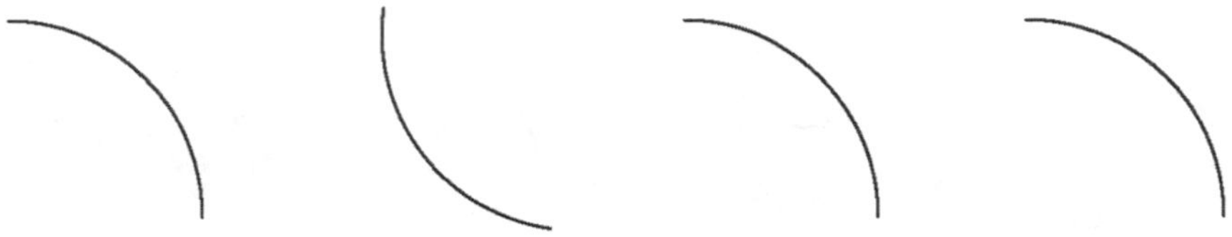

3

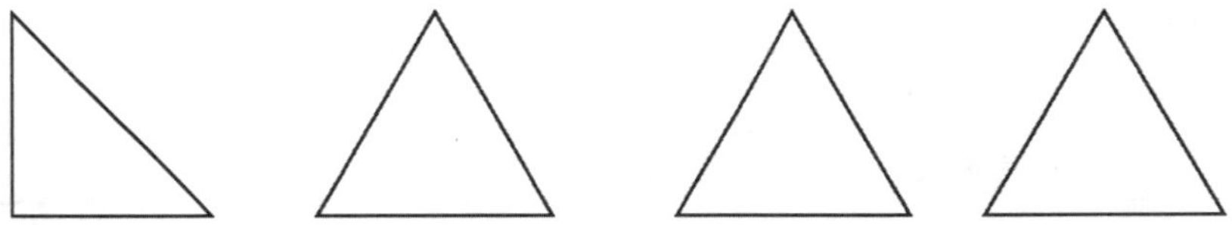

4

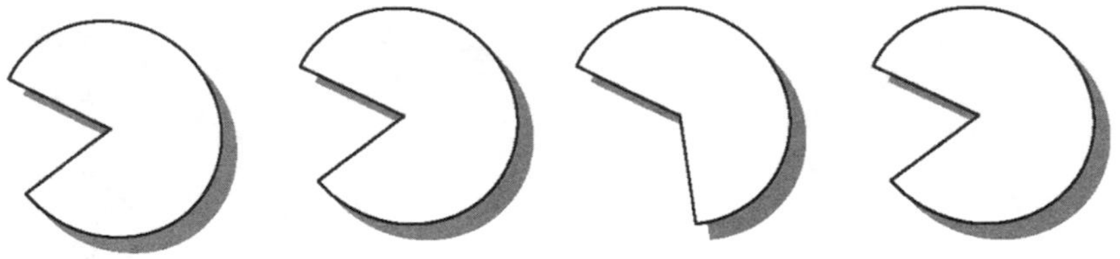

Which picture is different from the others?

1

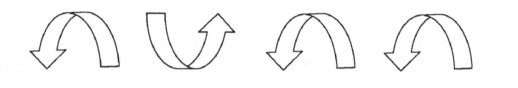

2

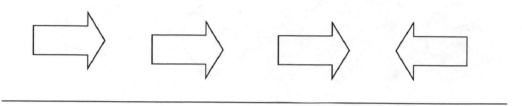

3

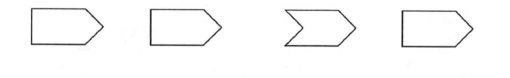

4

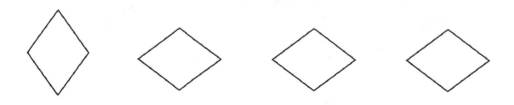

Match the figure on top to the figures below

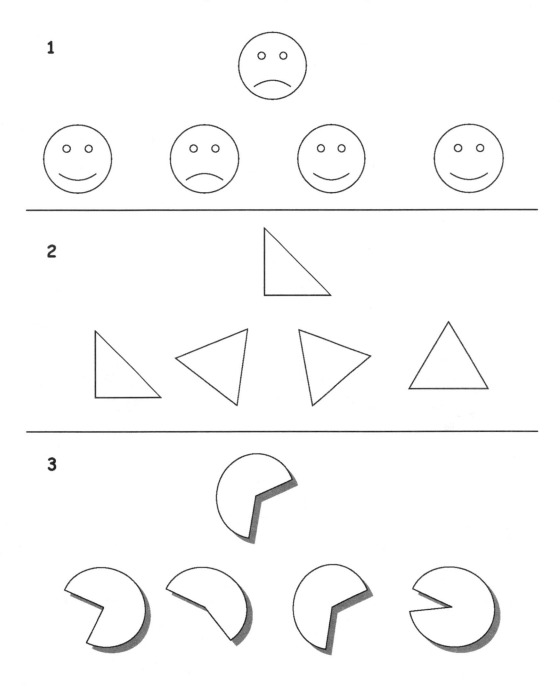

Match the figure on top to the figures below

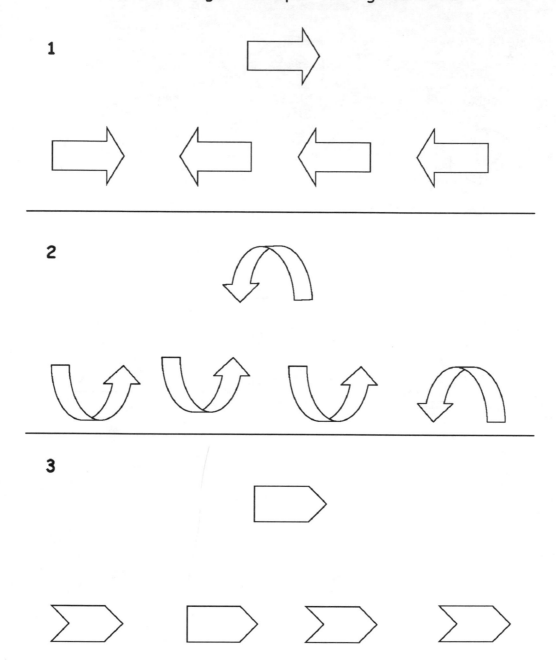

Match the figure on top to the figures below

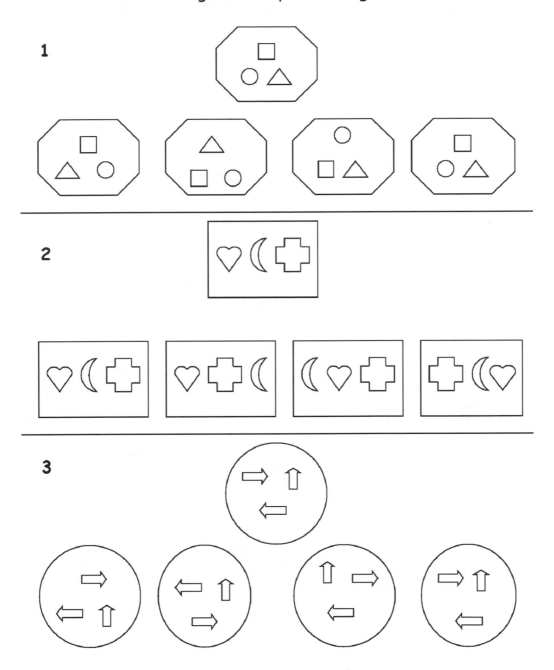

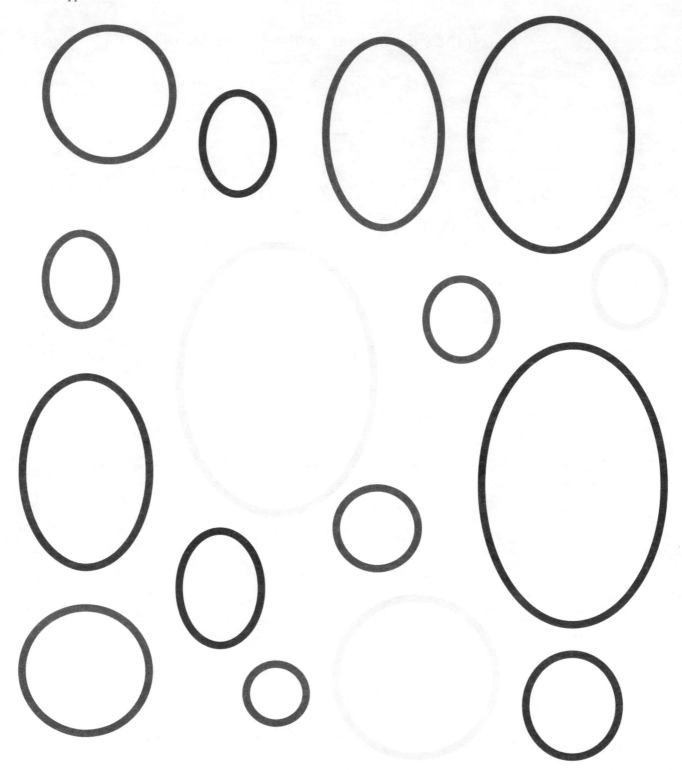

*Trace over circles with colored markers or crayons and then
use dot markers to make dots in corresponding circles.

Circle all of the letter "S"s in the picture below:

s   S   q   S   g   S   d   P   q
  d   d   s
q   c   a   q   c
S   c   s   H   c   S   p   a   c   S   H
  a   D   d   d   a   G   d   c   S   c   H   s   c   q

Circle all of the letter "C"s in the picture below:

e   l   E   C   c   c   c   C   L   e
      L   F   I   c   L   c
  c   H   F   e   C   C   F   H   H
C   I   c   I   c   c   e   E   H   c   c   F   C

Circle all of the letter "P"s in the picture below:

P   E   L   T   c   P   P   c   c   P   T   L
  L   E   F   p   F   E   h   E   I   P   p
          h   J   F
F   c   p   c   P   H   H   c   E   c   L   T

Circle all of the letter "J"s in the picture below:

j   i   E   J   F   J   j   j   C   L   j
L   H   I   I   L   C
J   F   e   J   j   F   H   H
J   I   J   I   c   j   e   E   H   c   j   F   J

Circle all of the letter "A"s in the picture below:

a   A   q   A   g   A   q   P   a   q
d   d   a   C
q   C   A   q   c   P   a   q   C   A   H
A   c   a   H   c
a   D   A   d   a   G   d   c   A   C   H   a   C   q

Circle all of the letter "Y"s in the picture below:

Y   E   L   T   c   y   y   c   c   y   T   L
L   E   F   y   F   E   Y   E   I   y   Y
y   J   F
F   c   y   c   Y   y   Y   c   E   c   L   T

Find the letter on the top in the figures below

1 A

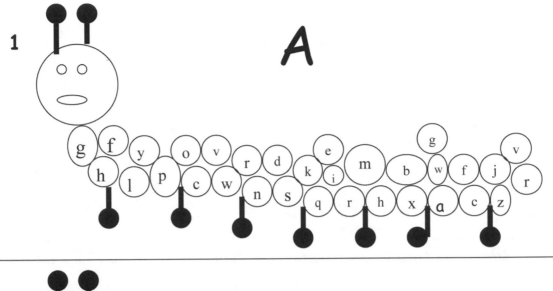

2 Z

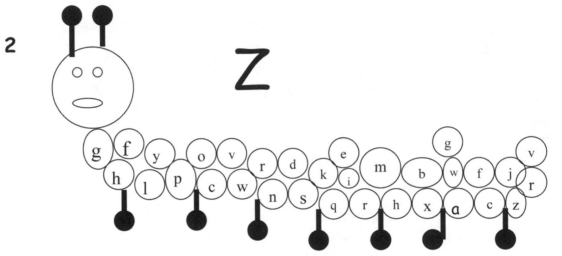

3 P

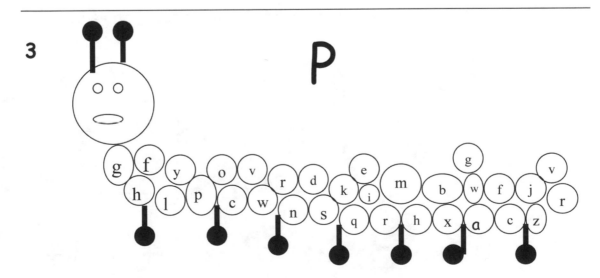

How many times does the number 17 appear in the picture below:

17   7   1   7   17   7   17   7   7
    2   17   9
    2   2   9   12   71
7   3   71   6   9   17   71   4   1   15   17
                    0   2
82   17   4   5   G   0   7   8   17   4   9   17
            7   17   17   8

How many times does the number 5 appear in the picture below:

5   2   8   5   5   5   5   2   7   5
        4   65   22   18   11
    5   9   25
            10   7   5   6   7   22   54
5   7   5
            58   5   1   1   3   2   2   5
                6   5   5

How many times does the number 34 appear in the picture below:

34   3   34   1   2   43   3   4   34   9   34
8   43   2
    4   3   4   43   9   5   3   4
                            34   8   8   6
34   9   5   0   3   14   2   34   4   0   14   11

Can you guess the hidden letters?

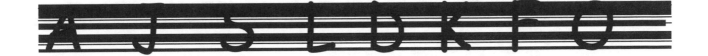

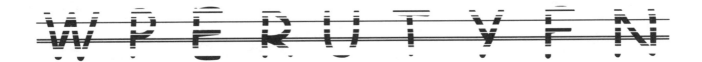

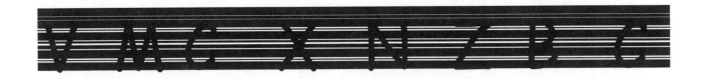

Can you guess the hidden words?

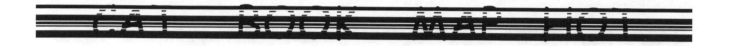

Match the complete picture on top with the choices below:

1.

2.

3.

Match the complete picture on top with the choices below:

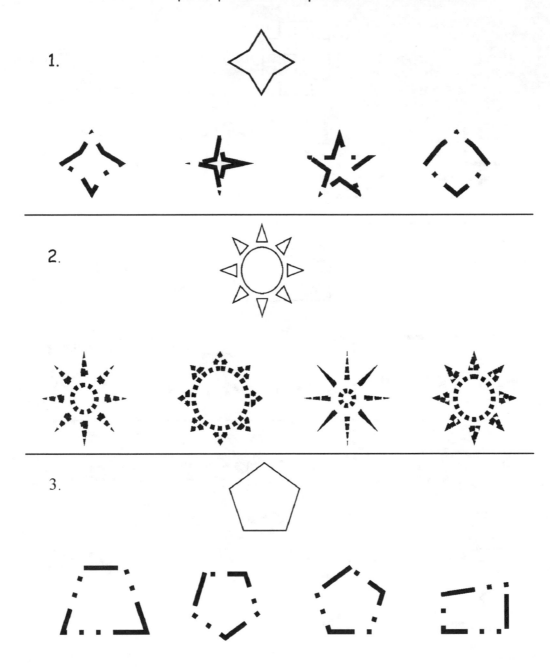

1.

2.

3.

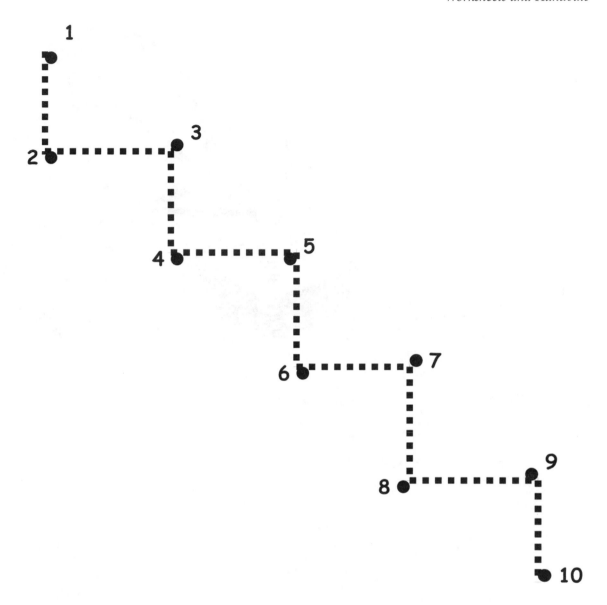

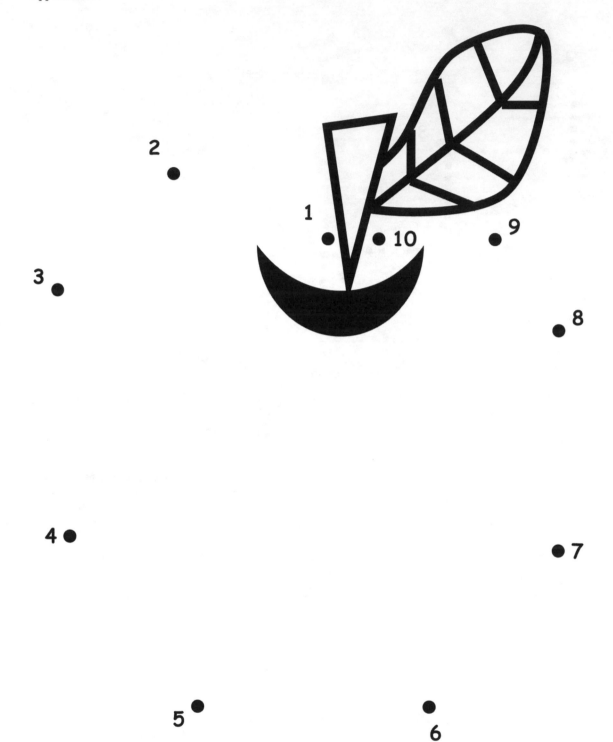

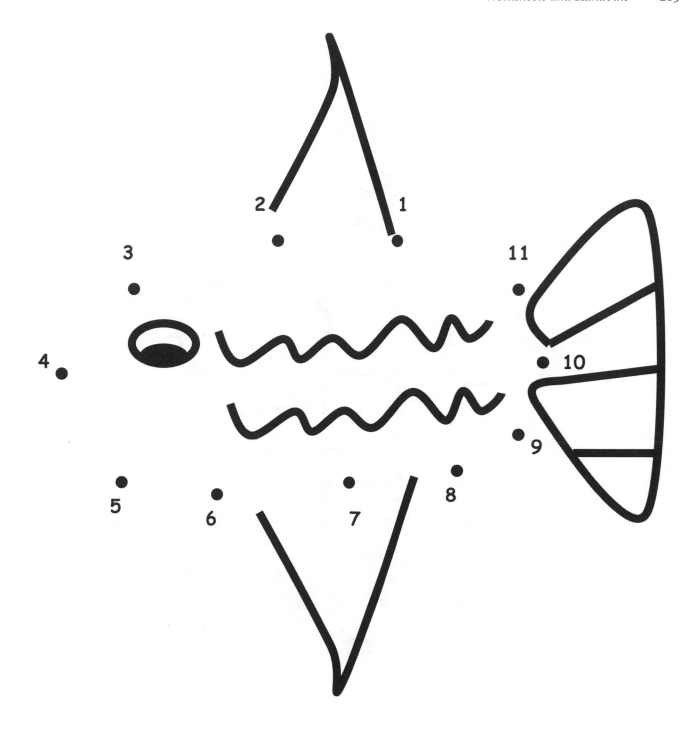

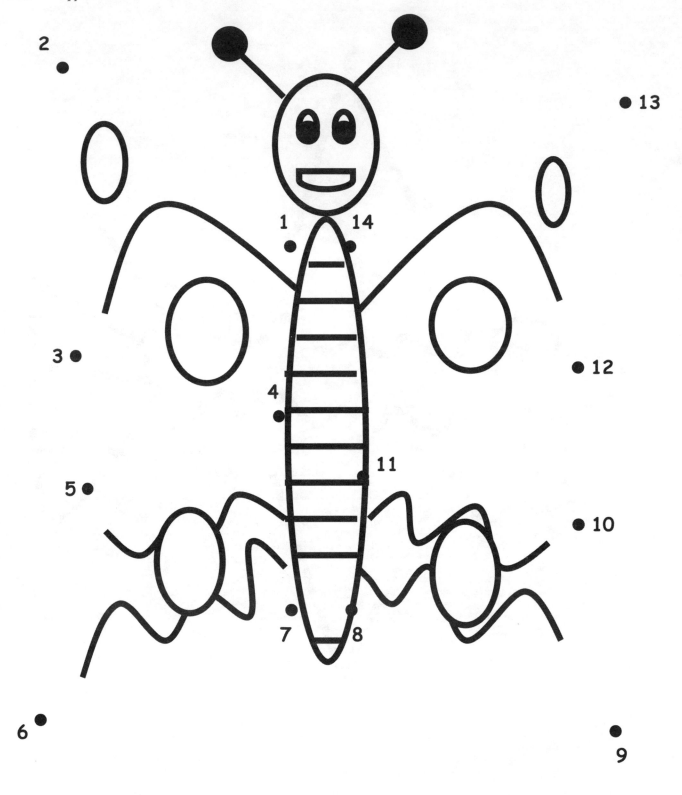

●
9

● **10**   ● **8**

11
●   ● **12**   ● **6**   ● **7**

13 ●

● **14**   ● **4**   ● **5**

15 ●   ● **16**   ● **2**   ● **3**

● **17**   ● **1**
▬▬▬▬▬▬▬▬▬

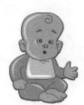

Help the baby find the bottle

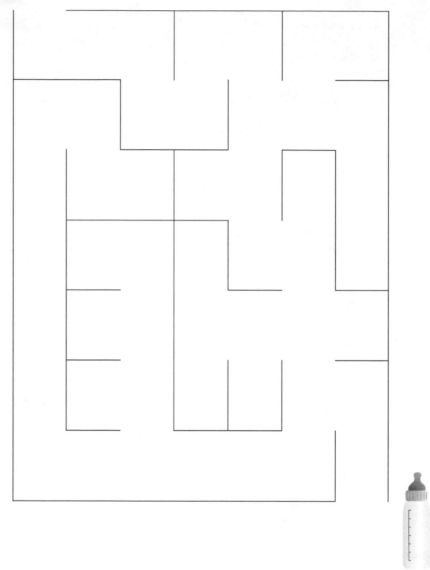

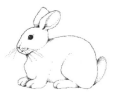

Help the bunny find the carrot

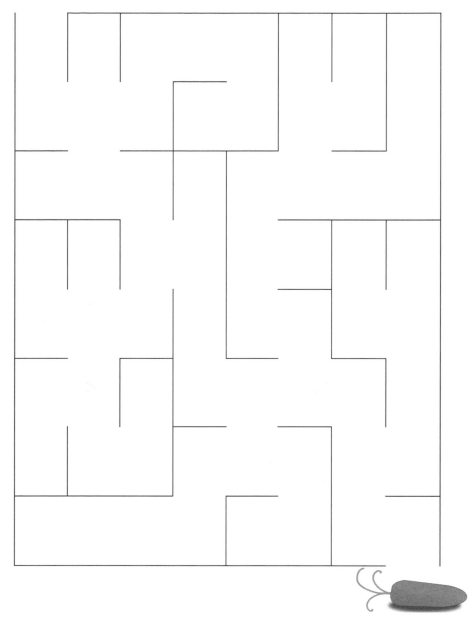

Help the dog find his food

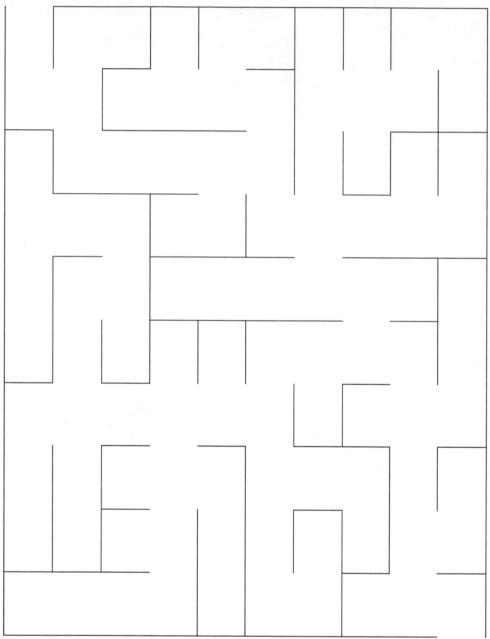

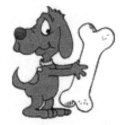

Help the bird find her nest

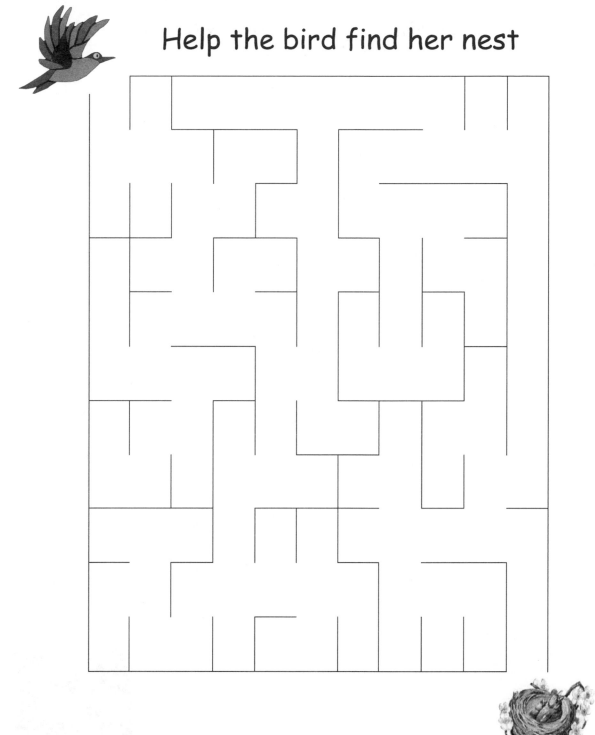

Help the magician find his wand

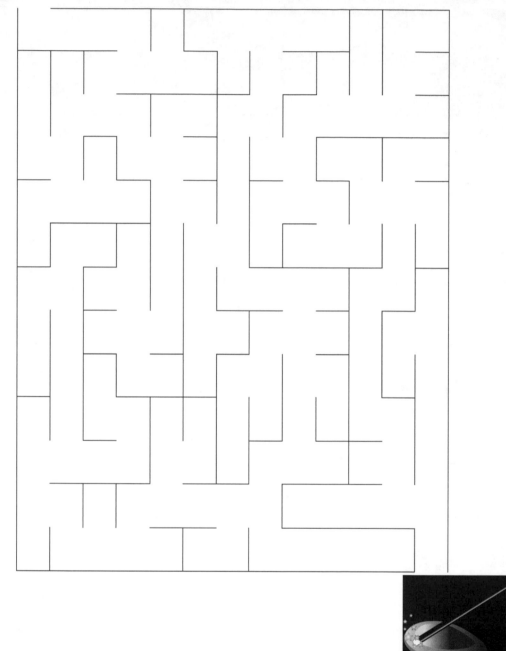

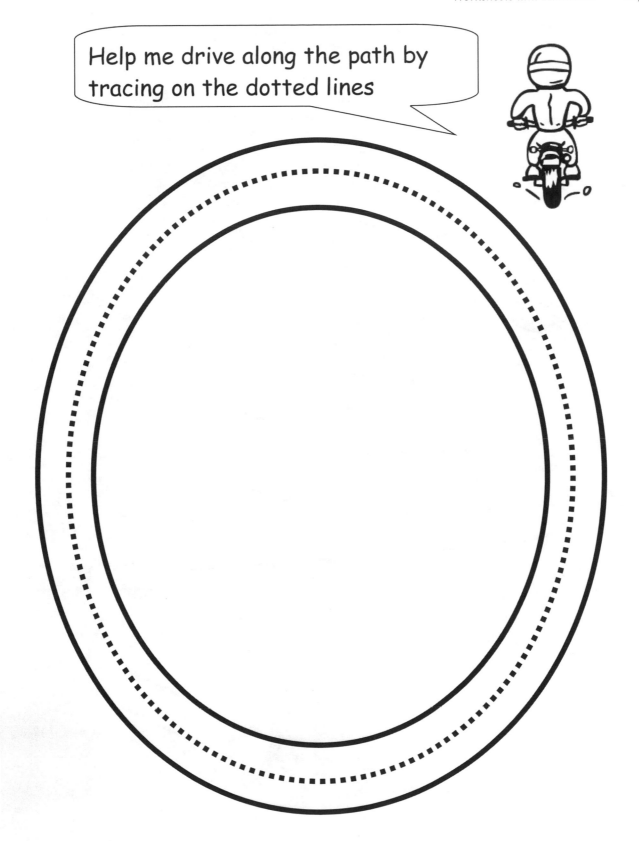

Help the man get through the jungle without bumping into the rocks or bushes along the way

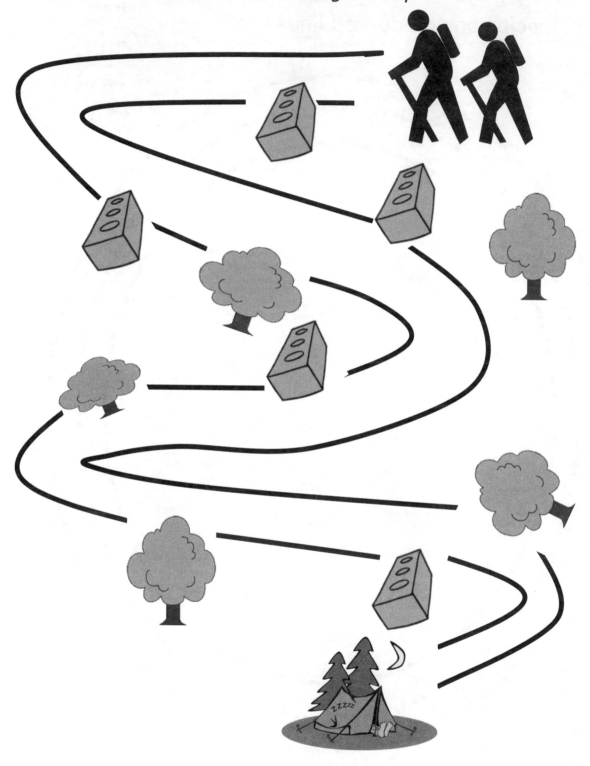

Help the school bus get to school by staying in the path

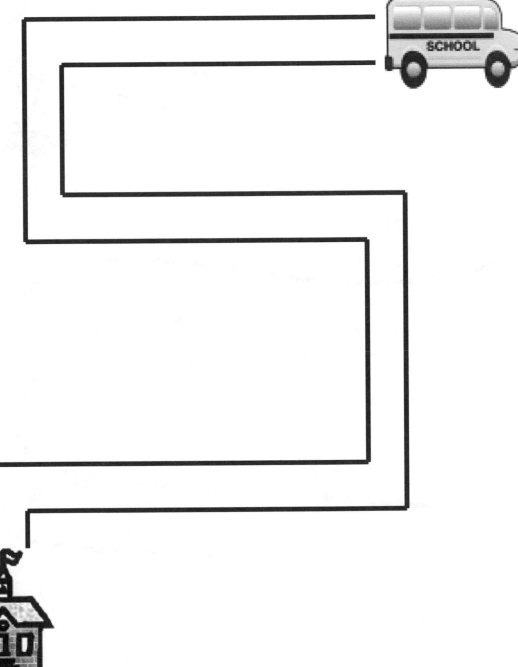

Help the girl get to the mountain
without going off the path

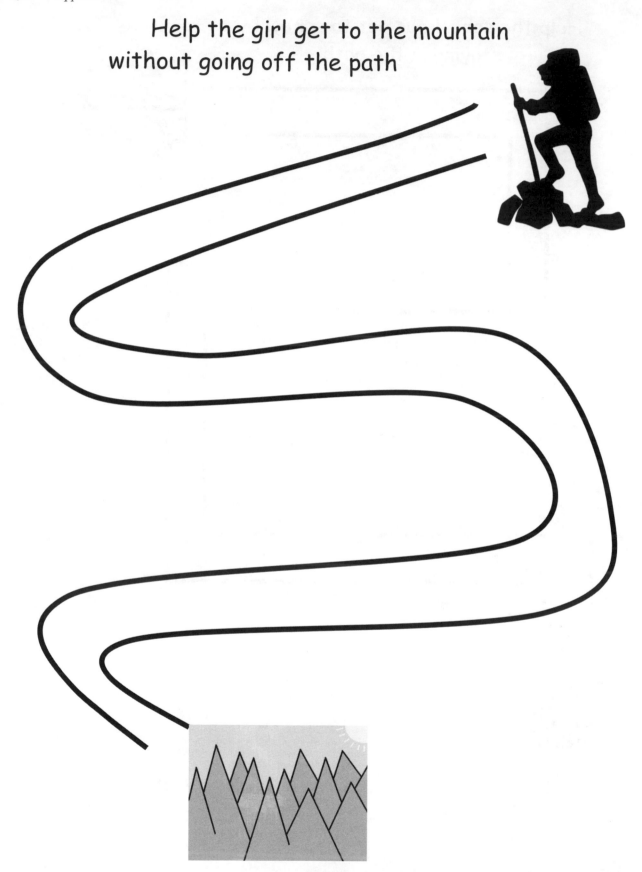

Help the birthday girl find her cake by staying in the path

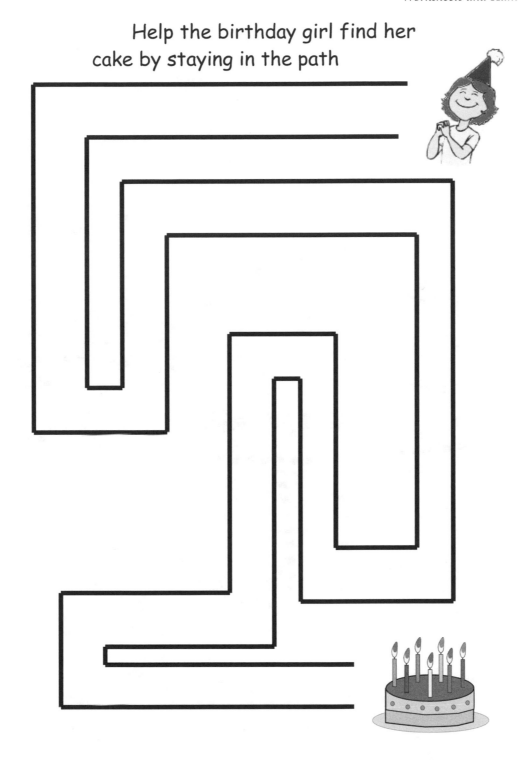

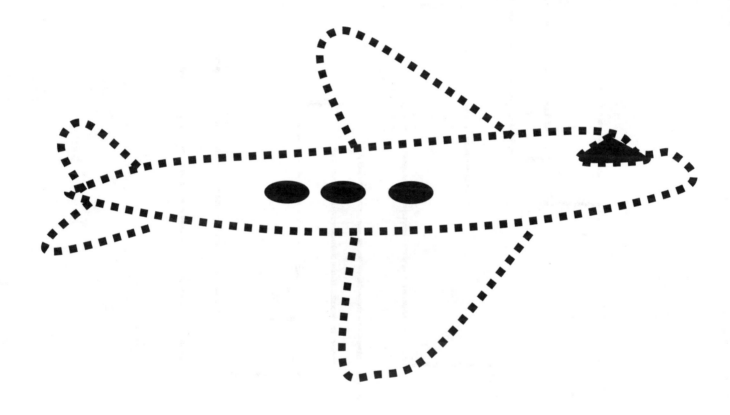

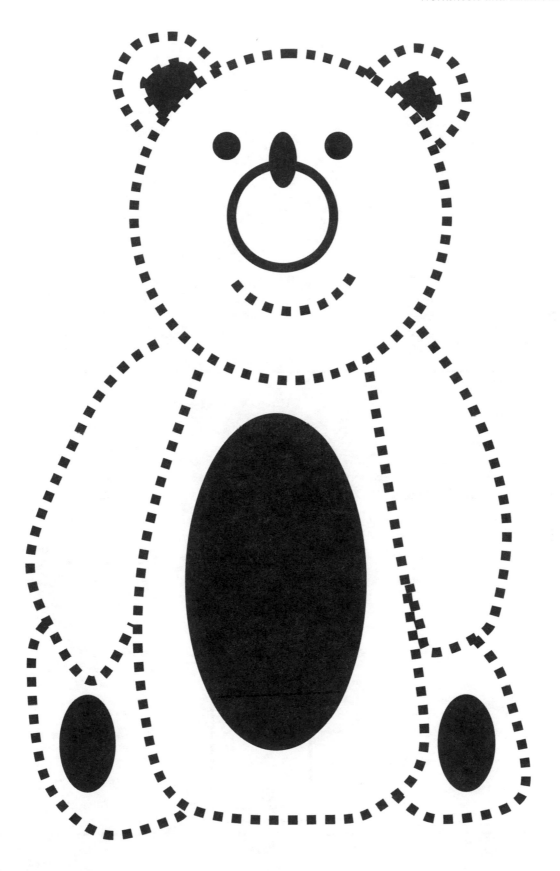

START

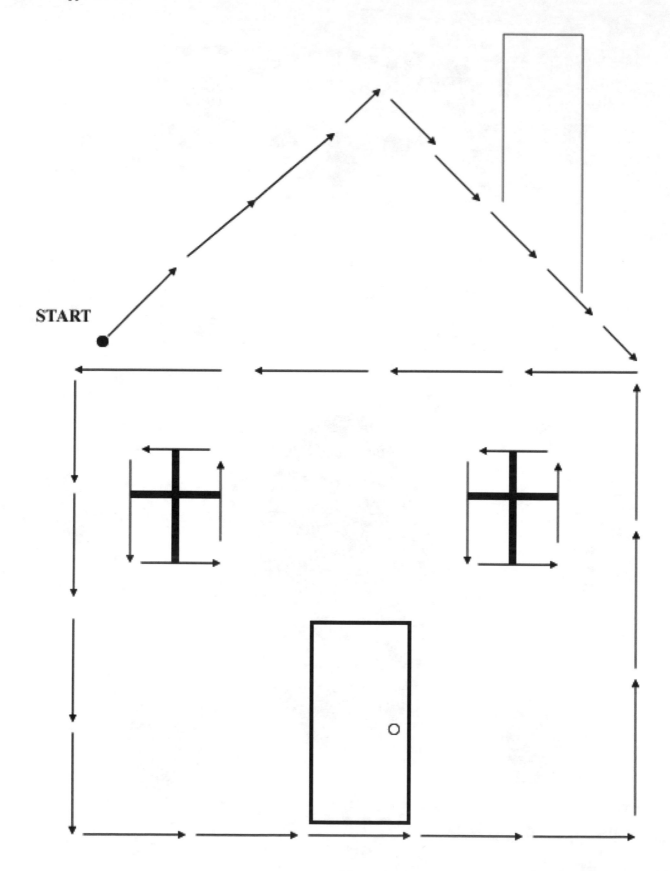

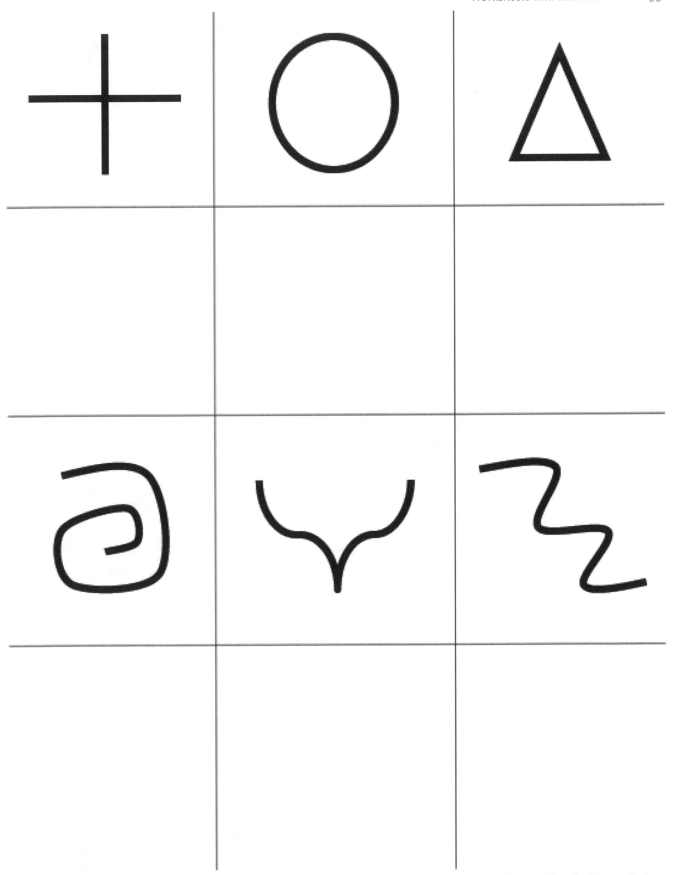

H	L	G	P	I	W	Q	U	S	A
D	X	Z	C	V	B	N	M	L	K
S	W	E	R	T	N	O	P	E	J
F	C	Q	E	V	Z	X	C	H	L
I	O	P	S	D	F	G	J	P	K
U	Y	T	A	W	H	B	F	D	H
H	M	H	Z	N	D	C	Q	M	I
E	H	B	P	H	T	F	O	H	E
P	I	O	J	X	H	H	M	G	R
H	X	F	C	E	G	J	A	M	H

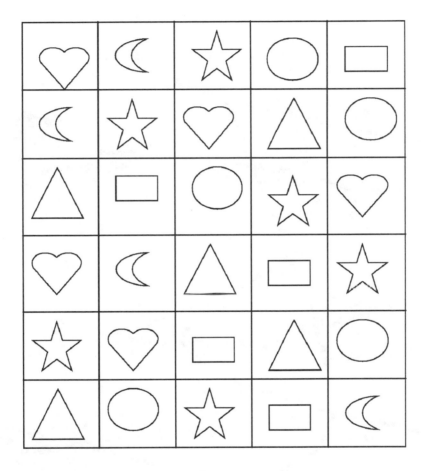

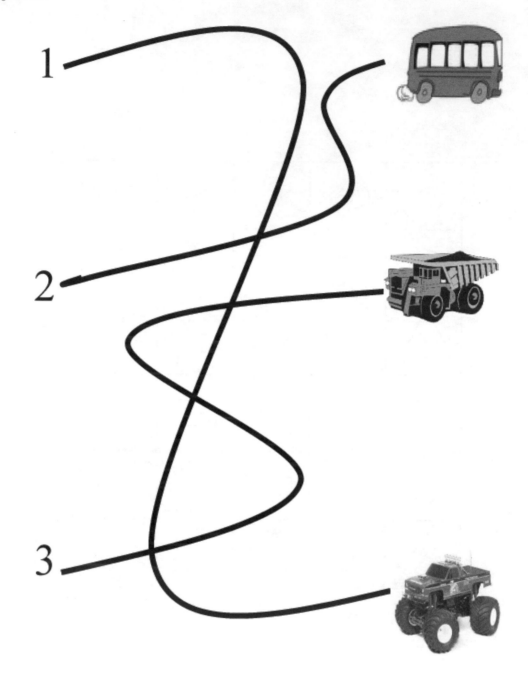

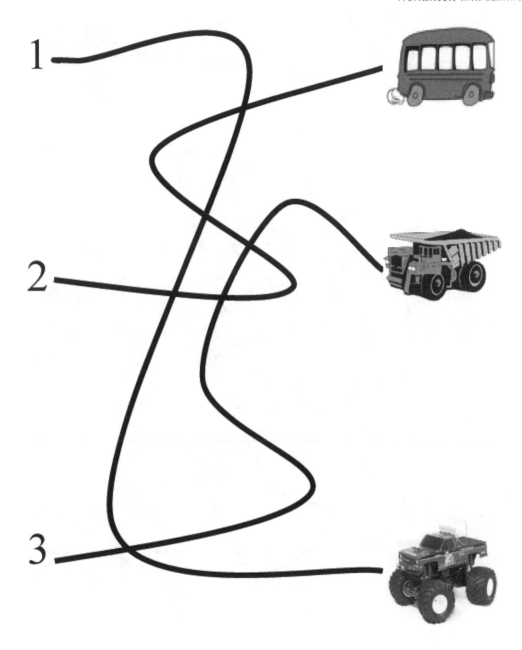

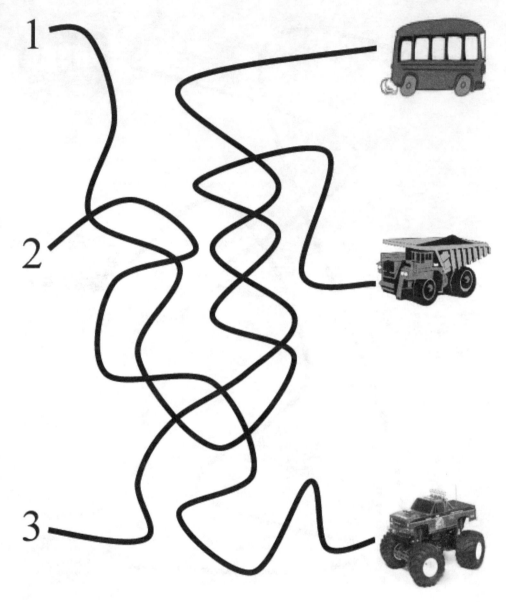

1

2

3

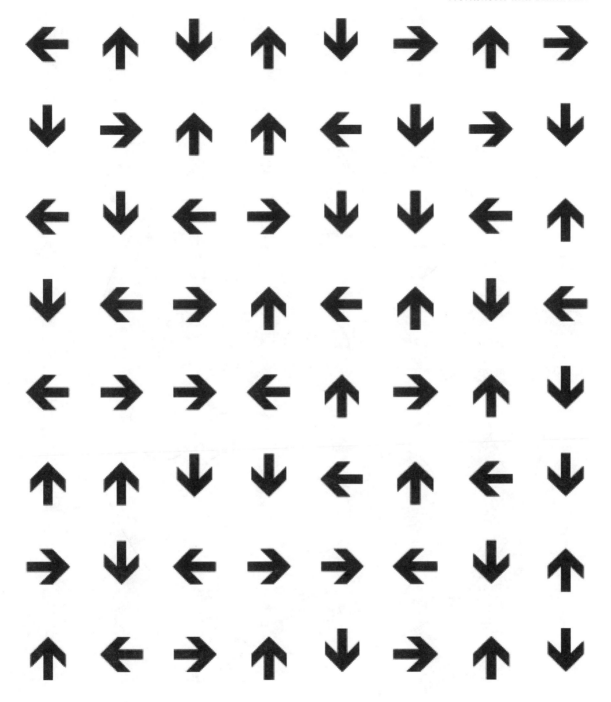

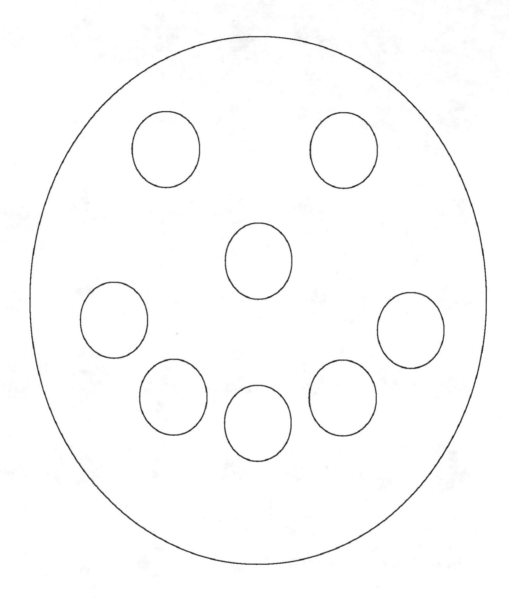

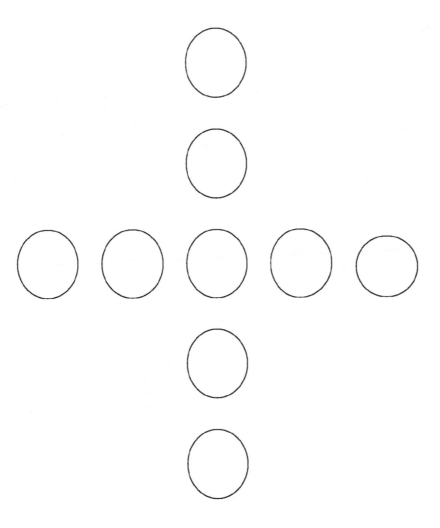

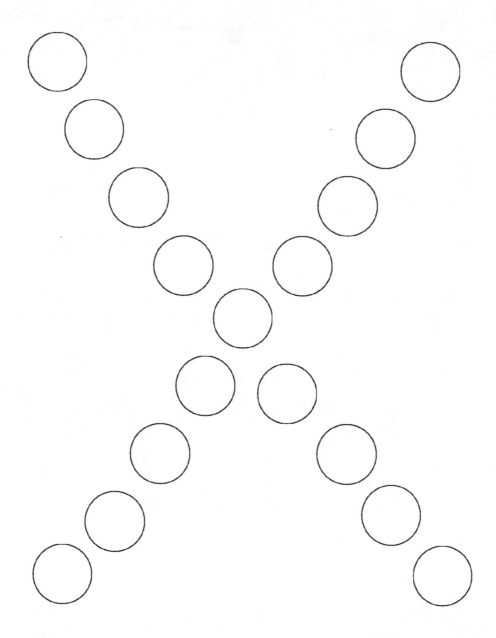

My Sticker Chart

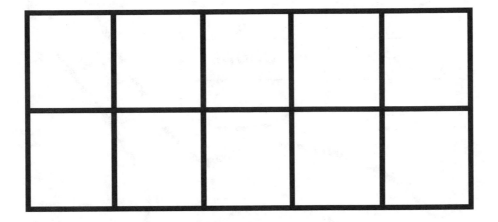

Y= Yellow   B= Black   R= Red   G= Green

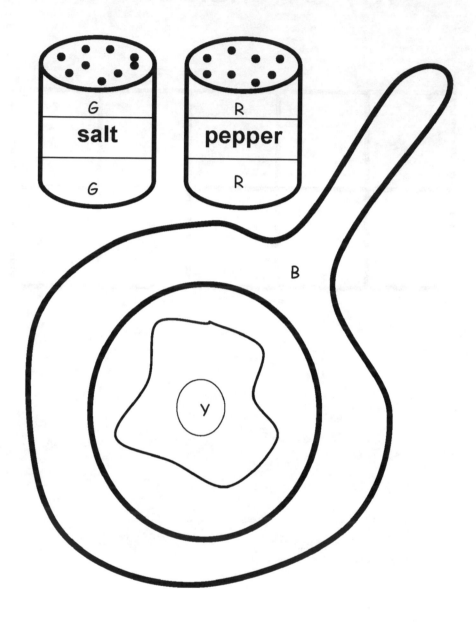

O= Orange R= Red Y= Yellow   G=Green

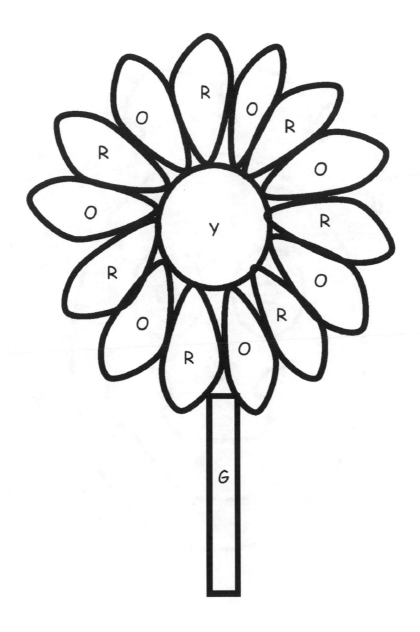

O= Orange   B=Blue   G= Green   R= Red

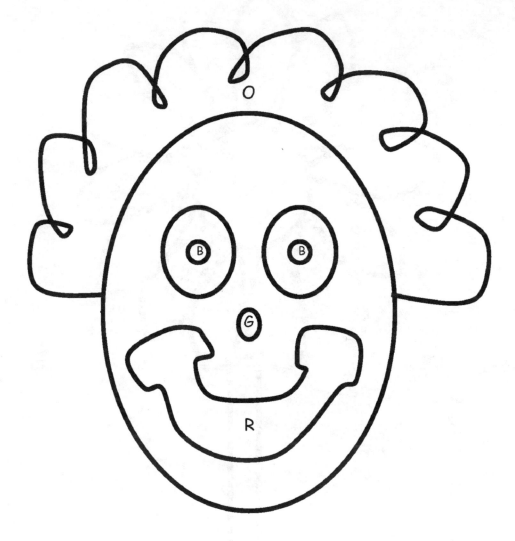

R= Red   O= Orange   Y=Yellow   G=Green   B=Brown

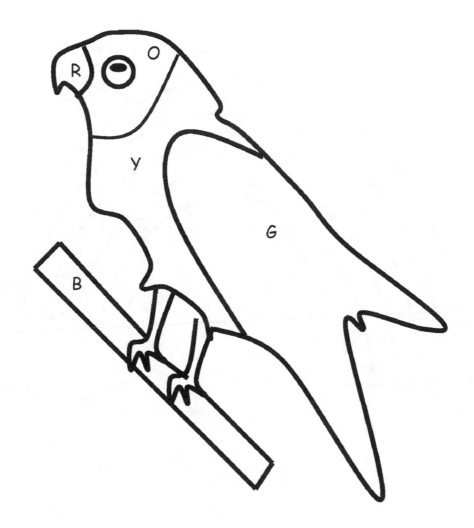

R= Red   Y=Yellow   O= Orange   B= Blue   G= Green

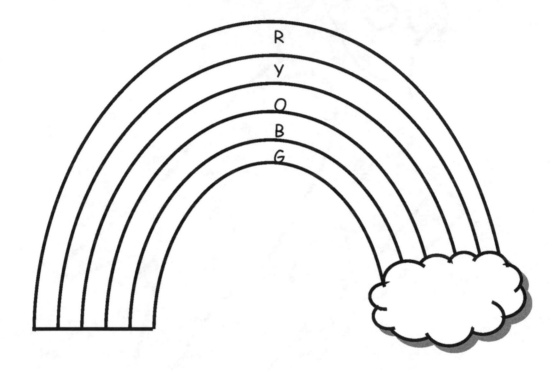

B= Brown   P=Pink   O=Orange

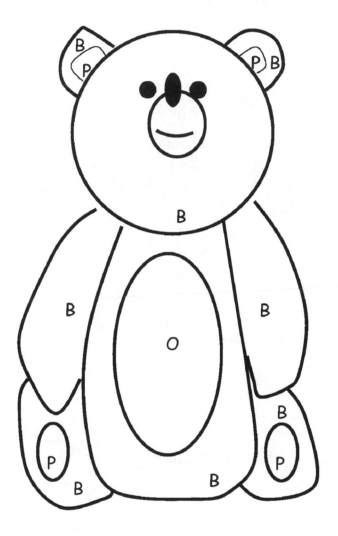

Scavenger Hunt

Can you find something ...

Bouncy
Shiny
Fuzzy
Noisy
Cold
Big
Little
Red
Yellow
Wet
Sticky
Soft
Hard
Round
Bumpy

Number Chart

1	
2	
3	
4	
5	
6	
7	
8	
9	
10	

Follow the key at the bottom to fill in the shapes

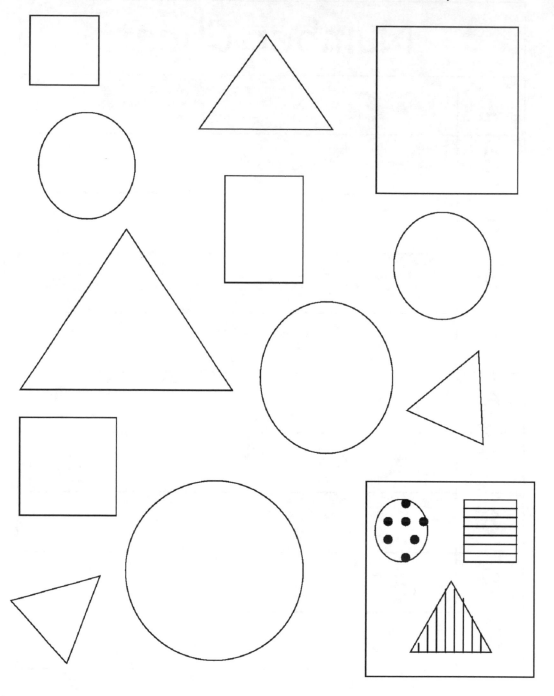

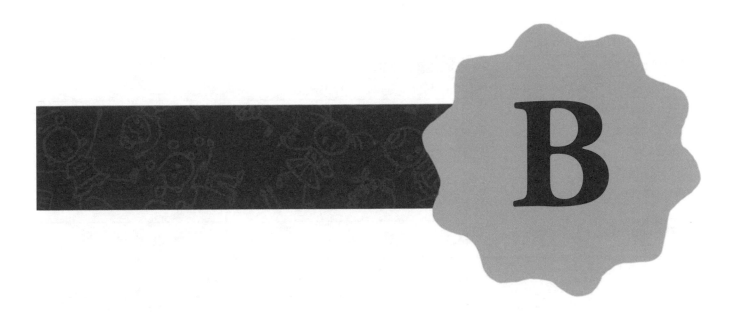

Therapeutic iPhone and Android Apps

To learn proper pencil grip, it is recommended to use a stylus, such as the Dano AppCrayon Stylus for Kids, with many of these apps, especially when working on handwriting skills.

SENSORY INTEGRATION	DESCRIPTION
Balance HD	Tilt the iPad to propel the marble through mazes of various levels (like Labyrinth game, but without holes for the marble to fall into).
Brainworks	Use this app to create sensory diets for kids at home and in school, etc. Comes with over 130 sensory activities.
Breathe2Relax	Instruction and practice of breathing exercises.
Dem Dancing Bones	Plays an anatomy song while skeleton dances. App allows one to select a specific body part and use that limb and joints to dance with.
Labyrinth	Tilt the iPad to propel the marble through the maze without letting it fall into the holes along the way.
Move Like Me	Imitate a sequence of dance moves while adding another dance move to the sequence, building on what the last player did with each additional turn. This game can be played by one person or two.
Super Stretch Yoga	Super Stretch superhero character and real-life children teach yoga poses in a fun way.
Zones of Regulation	Helps teach children to identify moods and levels of alertness so that they can better self-regulate.

Danto, A. H., & Pruzansky, M. *1001 Pediatric Treatment Activities: Creative Ideas for Therapy Sessions, Third Edition* (pp. 255-260).
© 2023 SLACK Incorporated.

VISUAL SYSTEM	DESCRIPTION
123 Glow	Color by letters and numbers.
ABC Coloring Book	Coloring page for each letter of the alphabet.
ABC Cursive	Letter formation of cursive letters to write cursive words and sentences.
ABC Draw	Fun app for practicing writing letters and coloring.
ABC My Little Farm—Dot to Dot	Connect the dots in ABC order to see the farm animal.
ABC Tracer	Teaches proper letter formation. Provides fun feedback of correct or incorrect strokes. Also includes words and numbers.
Action Potato	Game in which balls are thrown and player needs to catch them in designated can.
Balance HD	Tilt the iPad to propel the marble through mazes of various levels (like Labyrinth game, but without holes for the marble to fall into).
Button Board	Game that includes pictures to be completed by dragging the proper color-matched button from a tray of buttons to the appropriate place on the picture.
Cookie Doodle	Complete all the steps to bake and decorate virtual cookies.
Dem Dancing Bones	Plays an anatomy song while skeleton dances. App allows one to select a specific body part and use that limb and joints to dance with.
Dexteria and Dexteria Junior	Three activities for developing fine motor skills—tapping, pinching, and writing.
Dot-to-Dot Numbers and Letters	Dot-to-dot game with different age levels.
Count Money!	Practice counting money. For all ages. Various levels of difficulty.
Handwriting Without Tears Wet Dry Try	Simulates chalkboard to practice letter formation with the Handwriting Without Tears method.
Highlights Hidden Pictures Puzzles	Hidden picture game. When object is found, it turns to color and makes a sound.
iLuv Drawing Animals (and other iLuv Drawing apps)	Learn to draw animals by tracing over step-by-step templates.
iSays Memory Game	Simon game—tap lights in the same sequence that they lit up.
Labyrinth	Tilt the iPad to propel the marble through the maze without letting it fall into the holes along the way.
Little Things	A seek-and-find game where the player searches for a list of objects embedded in colorful collages made of thousands of "little things."
My First Tangrams	Copy a picture or pattern using the shapes provided. Have fun completing existing tangrams or creating your own. Rules are modified from standard tangrams to suit children.
Pirate Treasure Hunt: Eight Challenges	Child helps a pirate solve eight problems (e.g., math, reading, time, shapes, sequencing) in order to find the hidden treasure.
Rain Dots	Different colored dots rain down on the screen. Player tries to pop the colored dots that match the dots displayed at the bottom of the screen.
Rush Hour	As in the real game, player needs to get a certain car out of a traffic jam by moving other cars blocking the exit (varying levels of difficulty).
Shape Builder	Hundreds of fun, colorful, simple jigsaw puzzles at the preschool level.

Skywrite	Fun way to practice handwriting by "writing in the sky." Child can send message in the sky to a friend.
Write My Name	Children practice writing their names, tracing letters, and writing familiar sight words.
DISSOCIATION ACTIVITIES	DESCRIPTION
123 Glow	Color by letters and numbers.
ABCheese	Game where child traces a letter by moving a mouse to eat the cheese.
ABC Coloring Book	Coloring page for each letter of the alphabet.
ABC Cursive	Letter formation of cursive letters to write cursive words and sentences.
ABC My Little Farm—Dot to Dot	Connect the dots in ABC order to see the farm animal.
ABC Tracer	Teaches proper letter formation. Provides fun feedback of correct or incorrect strokes. Also includes words and numbers.
Action Potato	Game in which balls are thrown and player needs to catch them in designated can.
Balance HD	Tilt the iPad to propel the marble through mazes of various levels (like Labyrinth game but without holes for the marble to fall into).
Button Board	Game that includes pictures to be completed by dragging the proper color-matched button from a tray of buttons to the appropriate place on the picture.
Cookie Doodle	Complete all the steps to bake and decorate virtual cookies.
Dem Dancing Bones	Plays an anatomy song while skeleton dances. App allows one to select a specific body part and use that limb and joints to dance with.
Dexteria and Dexteria Junior	Three activities for developing fine motor skills—tapping, pinching, and writing.
Dot-to-Dot Numbers and Letters	Dot-to-dot game with different age levels.
Count Money!	Practice counting money. For all ages. Various levels of difficulty.
Handwriting Without Tears Wet Dry Try	Simulates chalkboard to practice letter formation with the Handwriting Without Tears method.
Highlights Hidden Pictures Puzzles	Hidden picture game. When object is found, it turns to color and makes a sound.
iLuv Drawing Animals (and other iLuv Drawing apps)	Learn to draw animals by tracing over step-by-step templates.
iSays Memory Game	Simon game—tap lights in the same sequence that they lit up.
Little Things	A seek-and-find game where the player searches for a list of objects embedded in colorful collages made of thousands of "little things."
My First Tangrams	Copy a picture or pattern using the shapes provided. Have fun completing existing tangrams or creating your own. Rules are modified from standard tangrams to suit children.
Rain Dots	Different colored dots rain down on the screen. Player tries to pop the colored dots that match the dots displayed at the bottom of the screen.
Rush Hour	As in the real game, player needs to get a certain car out of a traffic jam by moving other cars blocking the exit (varying levels of difficulty).
Shape Builder	Hundreds of fun, colorful, simple jigsaw puzzles for the preschool level.

Skywrite	Fun way to practice handwriting by "writing in the sky." Child can send a message in the sky to a friend.
Super Stretch Yoga	Super Stretch superhero character and real-life children teach yoga poses in a fun way.
Write My Name	Children practice writing their names, tracing letters, and writing familiar sight words.
HAND SKILLS	**DESCRIPTION**
123 Glow	Color by letters and numbers.
ABC Coloring Book	Coloring page for each letter of the alphabet.
ABC Cursive	Letter formation of cursive letters to write cursive words and sentences.
ABC My Little Farm—Dot to Dot	Connect the dots in ABC order to see the farm animal.
ABC Tracer	Teaches proper letter formation. Provides fun feedback of correct or incorrect strokes. Also includes words and numbers.
Action Potato	Game in which balls are thrown and player needs to catch them in designated can.
Balance HD	Tilt the iPad to propel the marble through mazes of various levels (like Labyrinth game, but without holes for the marble to fall into).
Button Board	Game that includes pictures to be completed by dragging the proper color-matched button from a tray of buttons to the appropriate place on the picture.
Cookie Doodle	Complete all the steps to bake and decorate virtual cookies.
Count Money!	Practice counting money. For all ages. Various levels of difficulty.
Dexteria and Dexteria Junior	Three activities for developing fine motor skills—tapping, pinching, and writing.
Dots 4 Tots	Children trace finger from point to point to create animals, shapes, letters, and numbers.
Dot-to-Dot Numbers and Letters	Dot-to-dot game for different age levels.
Handwriting Without Tears Wet Dry Try	Simulates chalkboard to practice letter formation with the Handwriting Without Tears method.
Highlights Hidden Picture Puzzles	Hidden picture game. When object is found, it turns to color and makes a sound.
iLuv Drawing Animals (and other iLuv Drawing apps)	Learn to draw animals by tracing over step-by-step templates.
iSays Memory Game	Simon game—tap lights in the same sequence that they lit up.
Labyrinth	Tilt the iPad to propel the marble through the maze without letting it fall into the holes along the way.
Little Things	A seek-and-find game where the player searches for a list of objects embedded in colorful collages made of thousands of "little things."
Mad Math	Adding, subtracting, and multiplication games.
Math Ninja	Action-packed game to work on math skills.
Move Like Me	Imitate a sequence of dance moves while adding another dance move to the sequence, building on what the last player did with each additional turn. Game can be played by one person or two.

MotionMaze	Help the pirate navigate through the treasure map maze by walking or jogging in place. The game is powered by child's movement.
My First Tangrams	Copy a picture or pattern using the shapes provided. Have fun completing existing tangrams or creating your own. Rules are modified from standard tangrams to suit children.
Pirate Treasure Hunt: Eight Challenges	Child helps a pirate solve eight problems (e.g., math, reading, time, shapes, sequencing) in order to find the hidden treasure.
Rain Dots	Different colored dots rain down on the screen. Player tries to pop the colored dots that match the dots displayed at the bottom of the screen.
Rush Hour	As in the real game, player needs to get a certain car out of a traffic jam by moving other cars blocking the exit (varying levels of difficulty).
Shape Builder	Hundreds of fun, colorful, simple jigsaw puzzles at the preschool level.
Skywrite	Fun way to practice handwriting by "writing in the sky." Child can send a message in the sky to a friend.
Super Stretch Yoga	Super Stretch superhero character and real-life children teach yoga poses in a fun way.
Write My Name	Children practice writing their names, tracing letters, and writing familiar sight words.
BODY STRENGTHENING AND STABILIZING	**DESCRIPTION**
Dem Dancing Bones	Plays an anatomy song while skeleton dances. App allows one to select a specific body part and use that limb and joints to dance with.
Jump Jump Froggy	Children jump around or have sit-up competitions with Jake the Snake. Game play is directly correlated with physical motion.
Super Stretch Yoga	Super Stretch superhero character and real-life children teach yoga poses in a fun way.
COGNITIVE AND HIGHER-LEVEL SKILL BUILDING	**DESCRIPTION**
Chore Pad	Provides child with weekly checklist of things to do. Child earns stars and rewards for completed tasks.
Cookie Doodle	Complete all the steps to bake and decorate virtual cookies.
Count Money!	Practice counting money. For all ages. Various levels of difficulty.
First Then Visual Schedule	Use images and sound to create multiple photo schedules of a child's daily routine to increase child's independence and decrease anxiety. Can use app's images or upload your own.
Highlights Hidden Pictures Puzzles	Hidden picture game. When object is found, it turns to color and makes a sound.
iSays Memory Game	Simon game—tap lights in the same sequence that they lit up.
Rush Hour	As in the real game, player needs to get a certain car out of a traffic jam by moving other cars blocking the exit (varying levels of difficulty).
Following Directions Fun Deck	Fifty-two illustrated picture flash cards with instructions to follow. Can work on single-step direction following or multistep.

SOCIAL SKILLS	DESCRIPTION
All About You, All About Me Fun Deck	Fifty-six illustrated picture flash cards available with "getting to know you" type questions.
Autism Emotion	App uses music and a slideshow to help teach about different emotions.
Bag Game	This app is a spinoff of "20 questions" designed to be played with others. Various levels of difficulty are available.
Between the Lines	Children practice interpreting vocal intonation, facial expressions, body language, and other social skills. App provides audio, photo, and video clips.
ClassDojo	Useful in the classroom in helping children improve problem behaviors. App generates data and provides positive feedback for desired behaviors.
ConversationBuilder	Designed to help elementary-aged children have multiple-exchange conversations with peers.
Model Me Going Places	Teaches children how to appropriately navigate various places in the community. App provides slideshows of children modeling appropriate behaviors at various locations.
Practicing Pragmatics Fun Deck	Fifty-two illustrated picture flash cards are provided. Children answer questions about politeness, problem solving, feelings, staying on topic, and other social skills.
SD "What Are They Thinking"	Sixty flash cards are provided to work on inference, reasoning, and conversational skills.
Zones of Regulation	Helps teach children to identify moods and levels of alertness so that they can better self-regulate.
IMPROVING GAIT PATTERNS	DESCRIPTION
Super Stretch Yoga	Super Stretch superhero character and real-life children teach yoga poses in a fun way.

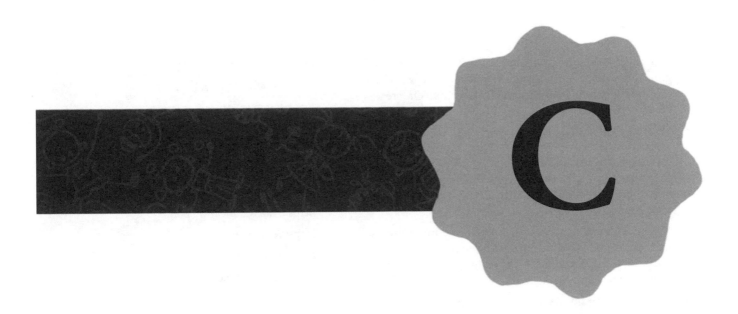

Occupational Therapy Telehealth

GAMES AND ACTIVITIES FOR TELEHEALTH

- Telehealth supplies scavenger hunt: Child looks around house for supplies (e.g., paper, crayons, scissors, glue, pencils) to keep in a box (can use a shoe box) for telehealth occupational therapy sessions.

- Freeze dance: Using Zoom or other platform therapist plays music. Child dances whenever the music is playing. When the music is shut off, child freezes until the music starts again.

- Simon Says

  ○ Therapist shares a YouTube video (e.g., "lets play Simon Says") with the child.

  ○ Therapist plays traditional Simon Says using various gross motor, fine motor, and stretching activities as the instructions that "Simon" is giving. Therapist and child can switch off being Simon.

- Picture schedule: Using clip art photos, therapist and child create a visual schedule for different sequenced activities such as toothbrushing, morning routine, recipes, or the schedule for the telehealth occupational therapy session.

- Digital coloring pages: Therapist shares screen of online coloring pages with child and child can color. (Can work on visual skills as well by having the child only color specific objects found in the picture.)

- Connect Four: Using an online Connect Four game therapist and child play Connect Four.

- Tic-Tac-Toe: Therapist shares screen with child and plays online Tic-Tac-Toe game.

- Sequencing activities: Therapist finds online sequencing games and shares screen with child. (Some websites with sequencing games include https://www.turtlediary.com/, https://www.education.com/, https://www.roomrecess.com/)

- Crossword puzzles: Therapist finds or creates puzzles online with crossword puzzle creator. Therapist sends child the link and has the child share their screen with the therapist. Child completes the puzzle and then writes sentences with the words found.

- Create your own word search: Therapist shares link with child and child shares screen with therapist. (There are websites that assist with this such as www.thewordsearch.com and many others.)

Danto, A. H., & Pruzansky, M. *1001 Pediatric Treatment Activities: Creative Ideas for Therapy Sessions, Third Edition* (pp. 261-264).
© 2023 SLACK Incorporated.

- Animal shape craft: Child cuts out various shapes and glues together to form different animals. www.crafty-beecreations.com sells templates for this. Or create your own templates.

- "What's Different" pictures: Therapist shares screen with child with two similar pictures. Child finds the differences in two pictures on the screen. (Some websites that have spot the difference games are https://www.hellokids.com/ and https://www.spotthedifference.com/)

- Mazes: Therapist shares screen of online maze games with child and child completes the maze. (Some websites that include mazes are https://toytheater.com/ and https://www.happyclicks.net/)

- Book scavenger hunt: Child looks at a picture book and finds different objects in the book as directed by the therapist (e.g., find a bicycle, a dog, something funny, clouds).

- Jamboards in Google Classroom: Therapist creates Jamboard and shares with the child to play games, color, or practice handwriting. (Jamboard is Google Classroom's interactive digital whiteboard; google "Jamboard for further instructions and sample templates.)

- "What's Silly" pictures: (Google "what's silly pictures" for many examples). Therapist shares screen.

  ○ Child works on finding hidden objects in the picture.

  ○ Therapist uses silly picture as a writing prompt in order to practice handwriting with child.

WEBSITES

- Typing
  ○ https://www.broderbund.com/mavis-beacon-teaches-typing-anniversary-edition
  ○ https://www.typingclub.com/
  ○ https://play.typeracer.com/
  ○ https://www.kidztype.com/

- Visual skills
  ○ https://eyecanlearn.com/
  ○ www.thewordsearch.com
  ○ https://www.spotthedifference.com/
  ○ https://www.highlightskids.com/
  ○ https://matchthememory.com/

  ○ https://mathsisfun.com/
  ○ https://www.digipuzzle.net/
  ○ https://www.roomrecess.com/
  ○ www.abcya.com

- Handwriting sheets, printables, and crafts
  ○ https://firstpallette.com/
  ○ https://craftybeecreations.com/
  ○ https://www.education.com/
  ○ https://edhelper.com/
  ○ https://kidzone.ws/
  ○ www.k5learning.com

- Educational/therapeutic games
  ○ https://papergames.io/
  ○ https://playtictactoe.org/
  ○ https://www.hellokids.com/
  ○ https://www.roomrecess.com/
  ○ https://toytheater.com/
  ○ https://www.wordgametime.com/
  ○ https://www.happyclicks.net/
  ○ https://www.primarygames.com/
  ○ https://shinylearning.co.uk/

YOUTUBE VIDEOS

- Movement
  ○ Shukla, P. (2011, June 17). *Stand Up, Sit Down Children's Song* [Video]. YouTube. https://www.youtube.com/watch?v=t9WAGkQUUL0

  ○ The Kiboomers. (2015, March 25). *Freeze Dance, Freeze Song, Freeze Dance For Kids* [Video]. YouTube. https://www.youtube.com/watch?v=2UcZWXvgMZE

  ○ Rocking Dan Teaching Man. (2017, April 14). *Do The Bear Walk (Gross Motor/Balance/Coordination/Self Regulation/Brain Break)* [Video]. YouTube. https://www.youtube.com/watch?v=KG3AO6lJ4BQ

  ○ The Learning Station-Kids Songs and Nursery Rhymes. (2014, May 18). *Shake Your Sillies Out, Brain Breaks Songs for Kids, Kids Action Songs* [Video]. YouTube. https://www.youtube.com/watch?v=NwT5oX_mqS0

○ incogneato72. (2011, October 11). *Bop 'Til You Drop* [Video]. YouTube. https://www.youtube.com/watch?v=3dXoiCMyyu4

○ Mitchell, D. (2018, August 21). *Yoga Yoga Slide* [Video]. YouTube. https://www.youtube.com/watch?v=bkhBtXah6N4

○ Mitchell, D. (2018, August 21). *Yoga Every Little Cell* [Video]. YouTube. https://www.youtube.com/watch?v=MPhgiyjNlUs

○ The PE Shed. (2020, March 22). *Teddy Bear Challenges—PE Home Learning Activities* [Video]. YouTube. https://www.youtube.com/watch?v=whPptTaKMtA

○ The Kiboomers. (2016, September 15). *Walking Walking Hop Hop Hop Song, Walking Walking, Walking Song* [Video]. YouTube. https://www.youtube.com/watch?v=r6cJB7k6eEk

○ Cocomelon Nursery Rhymes. (2017, October 3). *Head Shoulders Knees & Toes (Baby Version)* [Video]. YouTube. https://www.youtube.com/watch?v=QA48wTGbU7A

○ ChuChu TV Nursery Rhymes & Kids Songs. (2014, April 4). *Head Shoulders Knees Toes—Exercise Song for Kids* [Video]. YouTube. https://www.youtube.com/watch?v=h4eueDYPTIg

○ Cocomelon Nursery Rhymes. (2018, May 24). *The Wheels On The Bus* [Video]. YouTube. https://www.youtube.com/watch?v=e_04ZrNroTo

○ Little Baby Bum. (2015, June 3). *If You're Happy & You Know It* [Video]. YouTube. https://www.youtube.com/watch?v=vN_cgoVvsBI

○ Sesame Street. (2021, March 10). *Sesame Street: If You're Happy Know It Lyric Video* [Video]. https://www.youtube.com/watch?v=LDP08F3op80

○ Hartmann, J. (2017, December 15). *Exercise, Rhyme And Freeze, Rhyming Words for Kids, Exercise Song* [Video]. YouTube. https://www.youtube.com/watch?v=cSPmGPIyykU

○ Hartmann, J. (2020, September 1). *Crossover, Brain Breaks, Crossing the Midline* [Video]. YouTube. https://www.youtube.com/watch?v=RRlY1vWLS0o

○ The Learning Station. (2018, April 6). *Brain Break. Exercise Song For Kids. Fitness Songs Kids. Move With Me* [Video]. YouTube. https://www.youtube.com/watch?v=JoF_d5sgGgc

○ Hartmann, J. (2019, January 16). *Move It And Freeze Extended. Brain Breaks* [Video]. YouTube. https://www.youtube.com/watch?v=Nqg5zY0MOfI

○ The Learning Station. (2019, April 26). *Hokey Pokey (Original Version). Kids Dance Song. Brain Breaks By The Learning Station* [Video]. YouTube. https://www.youtube.com/watch?v=NhZI-ghmyrU

○ Hartmann, J. (2016, April 28). *Clapping Machine Is a Great Brain Breaks Song Engaging Kids With Clapping Patterns* [Video]. YouTube. https://www.youtube.com/watch?v=9sS0OeABaFs

○ Shukla, P. (2019, August 14). *Simon Says For Children (Official Video) By Miss Patty* [Video]. YouTube. https://www.youtube.com/watch?v=OkO8DaPIyXo

○ Hartmann, J. (2019, March 29). *Jack Hartmann Says. Following Directions Song for Kids. Brain Breaks* [Video]. YouTube. https://www.youtube.com/watch?v=OhRQSOMRk_A

○ Koo Koo Kanga Roo. (2013, December 2). *Koo Koo Kanga Roo—Dinosaur Stomp (Dance-A-Long)* [Video]. YouTube. https://www.youtube.com/watch?v=Imhi98dHa5w

○ Little Sports. (2019, October 3). *9 Min Exercise For Kids-Home Workout* [Video]. YouTube. https://www.youtube.com/watch?v=oc4QS2USKmk

○ Miss Renee OT. (2020, October 12). *"Mr. Bones" Body Awareness Online Learning Activity* [Video]. YouTube. https://www.youtube.com/watch?v=BccyyePMqsM

○ The Learning Station. (2013, January 9). *The More We Get Together—Kids Songs—Children's Songs—Nursery Rhyme—By The Learning Station* [Video]. YouTube. https://www.youtube.com/watch?v=lldmkrJXQ-E

• Emotions

○ Miss Molly. (2018, March 28). *The Feelings Song* [Video]. YouTube. https://www.youtube.com/watch?v=-J7HcVLsCrY

○ KidsTV123. (2013, August 27). *The Feelings Song* [Video]. YouTube. https://www.youtube.com/watch?v=UsISd1AMNYU

○ Learning Time Fun. (2016, February 3). *Learn Feelings And Emotions For Kids (Learning Videos for Toddlers)* [Video]. YouTube. https://www.youtube.com/watch?v=37w9JjUWN30

• Dressing

○ Flannery Brothers. (2012, January 19). *Dip N' Flip Jacket Song* [Video]. YouTube. https://www.youtube.com/watch?v=NpCNf4oTxg4

○ WonderGrove Kids. (2014, July 8). *You Can Dress Yourself S3 E10* [Video]. YouTube. https://www.youtube.com/watch?v=iugZbbUvAmI

- Fine Motor Strengthening
  - The OT Toolbox. (2016, August 30). *Finger Aerobics* [Video]. YouTube. https://www.youtube.com/watch?v=3VpARNgbb8c
  - HooplaKidz—Official Nursery Rhymes Channel. (2014, March 7). *Where Is Thumbkin. Nursery Rhyme. HooplaKidz* [Video]. YouTube. https://www.youtube.com/watch?v=bRNDu3O2VQY
  - Early Years Emily. (2020, April 4). *"I Like To" Playdough Action Song* [Video]. YouTube. https://www.youtube.com/watch?v=BOLR3pQt8zg
  - GriffinOT. (2019, June 9). *Crocodile Snap Pencil Grasp Childrens Song* [Video]. YouTube. https://www.youtube.com/watch?v=N6kPcQSSsEY
  - Miss Sprinkle. (2019, October 15). *Playdough Finger Exercises To Twinkle Twinkle Little Star* [Video]. YouTube. https://www.youtube.com/watch?v=1JaF0mjG4e8
  - HeidiSongs. (2015, July 30). *The Scissors Song. Music for Classroom Management* [Video]. YouTube. https://www.youtube.com/watch?v=-Qwi0l29ppY
  - Twinkle Little Songs—Nursery Rhymes. (2020, January 31). *Itsy Bitsy Spider Song for Kids. Incy Wincy Spider Nursery Rhyme (BIG CITY!)* [Video]. YouTube. https://www.youtube.com/watch?v=dTHv15w09pY
- Writing
  - Bailey, M. (2020, January 26). *Where Do You Start Your Letters* [Video]. YouTube. https://www.youtube.com/watch?v=j6eLk7fDLCM
  - OT Closet. (2020, October 4). *Handwriting Warmups With Pencil. Beginner Hand And Finger Exercises For Kids* [Video]. YouTube. https://www.youtube.com/watch?v=gMpq7ql9fAw
  - OT Closet. (2020, November 22). *Brain Gym Warm Up With Emoji And Metronome. Fine Motor Exercise For Fingers, Hands. Handwriting* [Video]. YouTube. https://www.youtube.com/watch?v=Iatni_Jk9ks
  - 123ABCtv. (2016, April 2). How To Write Letters A-Z—Learning To Write The Alphabet For Kids—Uppercase And Lowercase Letters [Video]. YouTube. https://www.youtube.com/watch?v=vsue4unC7YQ
  - Kiddos World TV. (2021, April 13). How To Write Letters For Children - Teaching Writing ABC For Preschool - Alphabet For Kids [Video]. YouTube. https://www.youtube.com/watch?v=C7oebqj3PCY
  - Hartmann, J. (2021, September 13). *Let's Learn The Letter A* [Video]. YouTube. https://www.youtube.com/watch?v=t2MfGBsnyZM (*insert the letter you want to learn for individual letter video*)
- Mindfulness and Attention
  - GoStrengthsOnline. (2012, March 30). *Teaching Mindfulness to Children at Home and in Schools* [Video]. YouTube. https://www.youtube.com/watch?v=iBpEYa74w2Y
  - Fablefy-The Whole Child. (2017, April 11). 3 Minutes Body Scan And Meditation—Mindfulness for Kids and Adults [Video]. YouTube. https://www.youtube.com/watch?v=ihwcw_ofuME
  - Meditation Channel. (2016, February 13). *Breath Meditation For Kids. Mindfulness for Kids* [Video]. YouTube. https://www.youtube.com/watch?v=CvF9AEe-ozc
  - Cosmic Kids Yoga. (2016, October 3). The Listening Game. Cosmic Kids Zen Den—Mindfulness for Kids [Video]. YouTube. https://www.youtube.com/watch?v=uUIGKhG_Vq8

Glossary

Bilateral integration: The ability to use the right and left side of the body together to perform an activity.

Body awareness: A person's sense of where their body and limbs are in relation to the environment and each other.

Compensatory strategies: Strategies employed that help a person compensate for decreased strength or weak skills (e.g., wearing Velcro shoes when a child cannot tie laces).

Crossing midline: The ability to reach across the body with one hand for an object on the opposite side (e.g., reaching with the right hand for an object placed on the left side).

Dissociation: The ability to move different parts of the body in isolation from the rest of the body.

Finger individuation: The ability to use each finger in isolation from the other fingers.

Grading: The ability to make an activity more challenging (upgrade) or less challenging (downgrade) by modifying a task or demand.

Input: Providing sensory feedback.

Motor planning: The ability to control and navigate the body and limbs in a coordinated fashion in response to the environment and during unfamiliar and new actions.

Pinch grasp: Grasping a small object between the pads of the thumb and index finger.

Pressure modulation: The ability of the body to know how hard or soft to grade pressure when interacting with objects in the environment.

Prone: The position of lying on the stomach.

Proprioception: The system that controls a person's awareness of where the body's limbs are in relation to the environment and each other.

Quadruped: The position of being on "all fours" (on hands and knees) on the floor.

Sensory integration: The body's ability to take information from the environment, process it through the different senses, and produce an appropriate response.

Supine: The position of lying on the back.

Tactile system: The system that controls the body's sense of touch.

Vestibular system: The system that controls the body's sense of movement.

Brand Name Products

The brand name products mentioned in *1001 Pediatric Treatment Activities: Creative Ideas for Therapy Sessions, Third Edition,* are listed below, along with their manufacturer information. None of the owners of the trademarks of these products have endorsed the use of these products in the manner described in this book.

- Angry Birds Mega Smash (Angry Birds)
- Ants in the Pants (Hasbro, Inc.)
- ARK's Grabbers/Chewy Tubes (ARK Therapeutic Services, Inc.)
- Barbecue Party (Goliath Games)
- Barrel of Monkeys (Hasbro, Inc.)
- Battleship (Hasbro, Inc.)
- Bed Bugs (Hasbro, Inc.)
- Boppy pillow (The Boppy Company)
- Bubble Wrap (Sealed Air Corporation)
- Bug-Out-Bob (Toysmith)
- Bumpy Grip (The Pencil Grip Inc.)
- Button Candy (Necco)
- Candy Land (Hasbro, Inc.)
- Cellophane (Innovia Films Ltd)
- ChapStick (GlaxoSmithKline)
- Cheerios (General Mills, Inc.)
- *The Cheerios Play Book* (General Mills, Inc.; Lee Wade)
- Clue Junior (Hasbro, Inc.)
- Colorama (Manfrotto)
- Connect Four (Hasbro, Inc.)
- Cootie (Hasbro, Inc.)
- Cranium Hullabaloo (Hasbro, Inc.)
- Crossover Grip (The Pencil Grip Inc.)

- Dano AppCrayon Stylus for Kids (AppCrayon)
- Design and Drill Activity Center (Educational Insights)
- Digi-Piggy Digital Piggy Bank (Gift Depot)
- Digital Coin Bank (Royal Sovereign)
- Dizzy Disc (Sportime)
- DMFLY Pencil Grip (DMFLY)
- Don't Break the Ice (Hasbro, Inc.)
- Don't Spill the Beans (Hasbro, Inc.)
- Doodle Dice Deluxe (Jax Games)
- Dynadisc (Exertools, Inc.)
- Elefun (Hasbro, Inc.)
- Etch A Sketch (Spin Master)
- Fantacolor Junior (Quercetti)
- First Hand (R&R Games)
- Frisbee (WHAM-O)
- Froot Loops (Kellogg Company)
- Gator Grabber Tweezers (Learning Resources)
- 3D Feel & Find Game (Guidecraft)
- Foam Grip (The Pencil Grip Inc.)
- Geddes Kushy Pencil Grip (Raymond Geddes and Company)
- Guess Who? (Hasbro, Inc.)
- HandiWriter Handwriting Tool (Handithings LLC)
- Handwriting Without Tears (Jan Z. Olsen)

- Hi Ho Cherry-O (Hasbro, Inc.)
- Hip Helpers (Hip Helpers, Inc.)
- Hippity Hop (Gymnic)
- Hula Hoop (WHAM-O)
- Hungry Dog/Monkey/Bunny Motor Skills Game (Lakeshore Learning Materials)
- Hungry Hungry Hippos (Hasbro, Inc.)
- Hyper Dash (Wild Planet)
- iPad (Apple, Inc.)
- iPhone (Apple, Inc.)
- I Spy (Briarpatch, Inc.)
- Image Captor (Westminster Inc.)
- Innergizer (Soleeze Innergizer)
- Jenga (Hasbro, Inc.)
- Jolly Octopus (Ravensburger)
- Katamino (Gigamic)
- Kerplunk (Mattel, Inc.)
- KID K'NEX (K'NEX Brands, L.P.)
- Kinetic Sand (Spin Master)
- Konexi (Wonder Forge)
- Koosh balls (OddzOn Products)
- LEGO pieces (The LEGO Group)
- Lincoln Logs (Hasbro, Inc.)
- Lite Brite (Hasbro, Inc.)
- Lucky Ducks (Hasbro, Inc.)
- Lycra (Lycra)
- M&M's (Mars, Incorporated)
- Magformers (The Magformers Inc.)
- Magna Doodle (The Ohio Art Company)
- Magna-Tiles (Magna-Tiles)
- Magnet Express (Anatex Enterprises)
- Mancala (California Dreams)
- Marshmallow Fluff (Durkee Mower Company)
- Mastermind (Pressman Toy Corporation)
- Melissa & Doug Basic Skills Board (Melissa & Doug, LLC)
- Melissa & Doug Latches Puzzle (Melissa & Doug, LLC)
- Melissa & Doug Magnetic Puzzles (Melissa & Doug, LLC)
- Memory (Hasbro, Inc.)
- Mr. Mouth (Hasbro, Inc.)
- Mr. Potato Head (Hasbro, Inc.)
- Nuk Brush (Gerber)
- Ocean Wonders Musical Fishbowl (Fisher-Price)
- Operation (Hasbro, Inc.)
- Oreo Matchin' Middles (Fisher-Price)
- Othello (Mattel, Inc.)
- Pattern Blocks & Board (Melissa & Doug, LLC)
- Pattern Play (Small World)
- Peg Domino (Sammons Preston)
- Pencil Grip Jumbo (The Pencil Grip Inc.)
- Penguin Pile-Up (Ravensburger)
- Perfection (Hasbro, Inc.)
- Perler Beads (IG Design Group)
- Pick Up Sticks (Commando LLC)
- Picture Perfect Design Tiles (Educational Insights)
- Plastic Jumping Frog Toys (U.S. Toy Company)
- Play-Doh (Hasbro, Inc.)
- Playfoam (Educational Insights)
- Pop Beads (Cousin Corporation of America)
- Popsicle (Unilever)
- Post-It Notes (3M)
- Pustefix Bubble Bear (Pustefix)
- Rainbow Loom (Rainbow Loom)
- Rapper Snapper (Ellis Enterprises)
- Rock Em' Sock Em' Robots (Mattel, Inc.)
- Rush Hour Jr. (ThinkFun Inc.)
- Scatterpillar Scramble (Hasbro, Inc.)
- Scrabble (Hasbro, Inc.)
- SET (Set Enterprises, Inc.)
- Silly Putty (Crayola, LLC)
- Simon (Hasbro, Inc.)
- Skee-Ball (Skee-Ball, Inc.)
- Skip It (Hasbro, Inc.)
- Smart Snacks Mix & Match Doughnut (Learning Resources, Inc.)
- Smart Snacks Sorting Shapes Cupcakes (Learning Resources, Inc.)
- Soft Cushion Pencil Grip (Charles Leonard Inc.)
- Spot It (Blue Orange)
- Squiggly Worms (Pressman Toy)
- Stare! (Game Development Group)
- Stetro Pencil Grip (Rose Moon Inc.)

- Styrofoam (The Dow Chemical Company)
- Sudoku (Nikoli Co, Ltd)
- Super Catch (U.S. Games)
- Super Sorting Pie (Learning Resources)
- Tetris (Tetris Holding LLC)
- Theraband (Theraband)
- Theraputty (GF Health Products)
- Tiddlywinks (House of Marbles)
- Tinkertoys (Hasbro, Inc.)
- Topple Chrome (Pressman Toy Corporation)
- Triangle Pencil Grip (The Pencil Grip Inc.)

- Twister (Hasbro, Inc.)
- Velcro (Velcro U.S.A.)
- Where's Waldo? (Martin Handford)
- Whac-A-Mole (Hasbro, Inc.)
- Wiffle Ball (The Wiffle Ball Inc.)
- Wikki Stix (Omnicor, Inc.)
- Woggler (Elrey Enterprises)
- Wok 'N Roll (International Playthings)
- Writing Claw (The Pencil Grip Inc.)
- Zoom Ball (Goliath)
- Z-Vibe (ARK Therapeutic Services, Inc.)

Index